CELLS THAT HEAL US

FROM CRADLE TO GRAVE

A QUANTUM LEAP IN MEDICAL SCIENCE

by

Roger Martin Nocera, M.D.

Produced by Scottsdale Multimedia, Inc.

ISBN-13 978-1460930052

Acknowledgements

THANK YOU

A special thanks to my colleague, partner and dear friend, Dr. Neil Riordan, a brilliantly skilled clinician, a medical genius and a modern day embodiment of Dr. Edward Jenner - the father of immunology. Dr. Riordan is one of the world's most important medical scientists living today, is the person who taught me everything I know about stem cell medicine and who has done much to sow the seeds to important medical advance in this century, as did his famous late father in the latter half of The Twentieth Century, Hue Desaix Riordan, M.D. whose written trilogy of history's medical mavericks has inspired much of this book.

Thanks to Berkley Biddel, a retired seven time U.S. House of Representatives Congressman from Iowa, who graciously helped me write important aspects of this book. Berkley is a deservedly admired, tireless political advocate for important changes in legislation needed to improve the American medical system.

DEDICATION

I dedicate this book to my beloved son, Michael Dominic Nocera, a spectacular and proud Outward Bound graduate, and my loving daughters Stephanie Lee Nocera, a brilliant high school senior who drives cars now, and Meleesa Megan Nocera, our beloved youngest (an astounding young woman in her first year of high school), and to their wonderful mom, Zandra Stephanie Jennas-Nocera, M.D., a superb diagnostic physician and a sophisticated soldier in the fight against breast cancer. I also dedicate this book to my profoundly insightful nephew, Sean Donovan, to whom I go for advice on complex matters when I think that things are not what they seem, and with whom I can share an accurate and inspiring memory of my wise and beloved late father Dominic Richard Nocera and my wonderful and brilliant sainted old mother Antonina Patricia Ferro Nocera, who along with my dad inspired the reality-checked common sense intellectual approach contained throughout this book.

A special thanks to my dear sister Paula Nocera-Donovan who graciously and lovingly allowed me to write this book undisturbed in her wonderful cottage by the sea in Newbury Port, Massachusetts, even though I burned the rug in the living room with a cigar that I knew, she knew, David knew and Sean knew I was not supposed to be smoking in the house.

PRODUCTION
Cover artwork provided by Sean Donovan.

Editing and production services provided by
Scottsdale Multimedia, Inc.
www.ScottsdaleMultimedia.com

CELLS THAT HEAL US

FROM CRADLE TO GRAVE

A QUANTUM LEAP IN MEDICAL SCIENCE

Roger Martin Nocera, M. D.

Roger M. Nocera, M.D.

Table of Contents

PART ONE

CHAPTER ONE

Every Hundred Years

"History is not, of course, a cookbook offering pretested recipes.

It teaches by analogy."

Henry Kissinger

Roger M. Nocera, M.D.

An Introduction to Healing Cells

"In a time of universal deceit, telling the truth is a

revolutionary act."

(George Orwell)

Only two other seismic shifts in medical science can compare to what is about to happen in conventional medicine very soon; one occurred roughly one hundred years ago and the previous one like it, approximately another hundred years before that.

In 2003 a major medical discovery was made. For reasons I explain in this work, it is the best kept secret in medical science history. Medical scientists discovered the existence of a human healing system contained in our human bone marrow. These naturally produced Healing Adult Stem Cells (let's call them "Healing Cells" for our discussion) are the body's own system of replacing injured or dead cells. Replacing injured cells is how the body heals itself—how it overcomes the harmful effects of disease and injuries. Harnessing the healing effects of this new medical discovery, we set up offshore clinics and began treating patients, often with astonishing results. Let me share one of my favorite treatment experiences with you.

In October 2005, I was contacted by a stranger in connection with my position at an international medical biotechnology company, one of the first of its kind. He had learned we were involved in very innovative new medical therapies that were unknown to most medical professionals. Because he was a medical doctor I immediately assumed he was contacting us about treating a patient. That wasn't the case. The doctor himself was desperately ill and asking for our help. He was middle-aged and suffering from a serious heart disease that ran in his family. According to his doctors he would soon be dead if he didn't get a heart transplant. He had already watched helplessly as two of his beloved family members died of the same fatal disease. His own medical expertise left no doubt in his mind how grave his prognosis was. The doctor would soon be dead.

A normal heart ejection fraction is 55 percent. His had dwindled down to a terrifying 30 percent. He was half way to the end, and he knew it. He had spent much of his savings for medical expenses toward his family's fatal illnesses and he had long since been unable to practice medicine due to his own deteriorating condition.

The dying doctor rightfully dreaded a heart transplant because he knew it would be very painful, extremely invasive and dangerous, and would cost a quarter of a million dollars—that is, if a suitable heart could be found for him before he died. If he did survive a transplant he knew he would be subjected to long term dangerous and expensive drugs required to stop immune rejection of the foreign heart and he would face periodic heart muscle biopsies to monitor the tissue's health.

Although this particular heart condition was new to our treatment procedure, we decided to treat the dying doctor with Healing Cells because we knew it would not harm him (as it never hurts anyone), and that based on our success with other conditions it may very well help him.

We gave the doctor healthy, live Healing Cells, obtained from an unrelated afterbirth, following a normal, full-term delivery—and why not?— the baby was finished with it, and she was going home with mommy and the afterbirth was now considered nothing more than bio-waste that had to be thrown out.

It was then arranged for the very ill doctor to be given Healing Cells, which were properly processed under the highest, universally accepted safe laboratory medical standards. These cells were administered through a simple I.V. line and, of course, required no drugs for immune suppression.

A few months after receiving Healing Cells his heart ejection fraction started to go up instead of the inevitable downward spiral. That nearly never happens; but it was happening to our patient. We were not even hoping for that level of improvement. We thought success would be getting him another year of life perhaps, a little more time plus a little extra physical energy.

To our delight within four months of this treatment the doctor had recovered completely. He has now withdrawn from all heart medications, has normal heart enzyme blood profiles, has a normal cardiac ejection fraction of 55 percent, and is back practicing medicine and exercising vigorously. The cost: just $15,000.

His prognosis? Excellent.

Our doctors have been helping patients using the therapeutic capacity of certain types of natural adult stem cells, Healing Cells, to treat not only heart disease but many others, often with similar stunning clinical success. They have demonstrated significant success with multiple sclerosis, rheumatoid arthritis, type 2 diabetes mellitus, autism, muscular dystrophy, cerebral palsy and spinal cord injury. I know of approximately 500 patients treated with Healing Cells, and I am convinced that so many of them would not have been helped as much by current "standard of care" therapies, of which I am well versed.

I wrote this book to publicly announce that this critical medical discovery exists, but is being ignored by our ailing healthcare industry, to our collective, potentially grave human detriment.

Many believe that the current problems with American healthcare (crippling costs and low effectiveness) are due to specific bad behavior on the part of our medical insurance companies, or big drug companies, or huge hospital corporate chains, or doctors, or the AMA, or even patients. At its core, the real problem is not due to any of these.

I document in this book the true underlying causes of our spiraling healthcare costs and ineffective medical care, and likewise demonstrate how once our FDA stops denying our nation's capable physicians their civil right to focus upon it., then Healing Cell treatments will rapidly revolutionize healthcare in a manner that will reduce costs to a fraction of the current system and drastically improve the health of our citizens.

We and other Americans have done the initial work, inconveniently overseas, demonstrating "proof of concept" of Healing Cells.

Now the FDA must lift its embargo on this completely natural treatment and allow our learned American physicians to begin to offer this safe treatment and database their results so that standard treatment regimens can be established for each disease and condition.

There is much work to be done, but the rewards are enormous and could come to us rapidly.

Two Centuries Ago

"Look deep into nature,
and then you will understand everything."

(Albert Einstein)

It was the end of the 18th Century, a little over 200 years ago (1796 A.D.), when a country doctor named Edward Jenner had a flash of insight that would change the world forever.

The medical insight itself was brilliant, but equally extraordinary was the sheer professional courage that Jenner displayed when he actually started to use this medical insight to help his patients. All the while many of the local folks were saying quite emphatically that the good doctor was absolutely, certifiably crazy for doing it.

As a medical doctor myself I can confidently advise you that most physicians, of any era, are not really that big on being called crazy by the townsfolk since it rarely fits in well with their future medical career ambitions.

The insight started to form in Jenner's mind as he contemplated that country women who milked cows for a living, during that era, called milkmaids, were **not affected by smallpox epidemics** in the same terrible way that everyone else was. Two centuries ago smallpox epidemics were horrible. They were dreaded scourges, with 30-40 percent of infected victims dying an agonizing, painful death, and those "lucky" enough to survive the disease developed severe deforming scars on their skin, especially their faces, which they carried for life.

Smallpox infection produced skin blisters called "pox," which covered the patient's body and oozed smallpox germ-containing infectious, disgusting pus. Milkmaids seemed to be "immune" to smallpox, although Jenner did not have the modern meaning of the word "immunity" at his disposal to help him, because in 1796 the human immune **organ system** had not yet been discovered by anyone.

There was another infection that produced similar pus-oozing blisters, a disease that was also common during that era which people caught from touching infected cows. This disease was aptly named cowpox and also produced skin "pox", which likewise oozed disgusting pus.

Cowpox, however, didn't kill people the way smallpox did as much as it annoyed them for a while. Smallpox was deadly, while cowpox was a very mild disease by comparison.

Jenner realized that most milkmaids had the mild cowpox infection at some time as it was very common and could hardly be avoided by anyone in constant physical contact with cows. Jenner envisioned that the germs that produced the cowpox and smallpox diseases were very similar to each other since they both caused similar looking pus-oozing skin blisters. And milkmaids catch cowpox only once. So, the milkmaids' bodies were somehow "remembering" the first cowpox infection experience, which somehow or another enabled their bodies to resist a reinfection when exposed to the cowpox germ a second time.

Maybe, because both cowpox and smallpox germs produced similar appearing pus-oozing blisters, perhaps they are similar in other ways (similar pathogenesis reflecting similarities in pathogen structure and probable antigenicity).

Perhaps, Jenner thought, the cowpox and smallpox germs might be enough alike that once someone got sick with cowpox their body in some way or another became "immune" not only to the cowpox germs, but also to the similar, but terrible smallpox germs.

Wouldn't that explain the link between cowpox and smallpox?

That would explain why milkmaids didn't get the dreadful smallpox disease.

What Jenner was about to do next has been declared by virtually every medical historian to be the most beneficial human action ever taken by any person in all of human history.

Jenner's Next Move

Because of Jenner's key medical observations and enlightened epidemiological analysis, the innovative country doctor created his famous **smallpox vaccine**.

He created a smallpox vaccine for his country-folk patients within his little country doctor's office. An office that sat next to the old country barn, where the wise Dr. Jenner made scratches on this patients' arms with a surgical knife blade, then he proceeded to smeared someone else's disgusting, infectious, cowpox-oozing pus onto their open scratch wounds!

Of course, this freaked people out considerably.

Poor Dr. Jenner was severely, publicly ridiculed for doing this. Among many other insults hurled at him were the widely publicized newspaper cartoons, which all played upon the same basic theme, which depicted a crazed-looking cartoon Dr. Jenner with his cowpox vaccinated cartoon patients, pictured sprouting cow heads, with horns, and cowbells on their cartoon arms and necks.

They had hoofed legs coming out of their bellies and long cow-tails growing out from their derrières.

It was all very humorous.

This public derision remained brutally embarrassing for the doctor and bruised his medical confidence a bit … until the next merciless, earth-scorching **smallpox epidemic** came rolling into town.

Reality happens.

Jenner's purposefully infected patients (inoculated patients) remarkably, extraordinarily and historically remained safe from the smallpox disease during that smallpox epidemic. A bitter irony of this experience was that many who had scoffed at Jenner's efforts and hard work, the very people Jenner was trying to help, suffered, perished or lost loved ones, including their children, to the horrific and painful small pox disease. Dr. Jenner's story makes me think of my Dad's words to me as I was growing up … "Son, just because something seems funny, does not necessarily make it truly funny."

A paradigm shift
Immunology had been invented, facilitated by Dr. Jenner's discovery of **nature's** human immune system.

The amount of human suffering and death eliminated by the derivative vaccine inventions directly linked to this one simple discovery of nature (and Jenner's willingness to act on it) is unfathomable.

It has been repeatedly and accurately stated by virtually every medical historian that no other discovery and no other human being has so permanently improved human health and so profoundly advanced the human condition on our planet. The diseases currently controlled by the vaccine medical paradigm include: diphtheria, tetanus, poliomyelitis, meningococcal meningitis, pertussis, rubiola, rubella, Haemophilus influenza, hepatitis B, smallpox and viral influenza. .

> "Advances in medicine and agriculture have saved
> vastly more lives than have been lost in all the wars in
> history."
>
> (Dr. Carl Sagan)

Notably, the urban medical scientific literati and greatly admired medical science professors of Jenner's era (whose names no one has reason to remember now) ridiculed Jenner even after he had saved many lives because they refused to believe it was his actions that had saved them. They considered the Jenner cowpox vaccine idea preposterous. My God, this Dr. Jenner - a simple country doctor living and practicing medicine "out in the sticks" - logically could not possibly be correct about these outlandish vaccine medical stories.

They rejected Jenner's observations out of hand. They turned their backs on his great discovery and refused to focus research on Jenner's treatment regimen.

Of course, leaders and intellectuals in non-medical fields blindly followed these learned professionals simply because it seemed logical to assume that they knew the truth on important medical issues. Sadly, the medical error on this matter delayed for many the badly needed benefits that would eventually be realized from Jenner's work. This is factual medical history.

"There are two ways to be fooled:

One is to believe what isn't so;

the other is to refuse to believe what is so."

(Kierkegaard)

One Century Ago

Let's skip forward to 1928. A little over 100 years after Dr. Jenner's discovery, the next comparable medical event, in terms of the degree of subsequent impact on humanity, occurred when Dr. Alexander Fleming discovered something that had also evolved **naturally**, this time within a common mold (a fungus): a natural "antibiotic" reality, Penicillin.

Fleming received the Nobel Prize for his enormous contribution to humanity, yet, he insisted repeatedly, that he had only observed what was occurring **normally within nature**, quite serendipitously. I suggest that Fleming was not just being modest as was widely believed, but rather, scientifically, profoundly and precisely accurate.

Fleming knew he was being honored for a huge and unexpected contribution to the human race that was triggered merely by his keen observation of nature. He observed that certain germs (Gram + Staphylococcus aureus bacteria) would not grow within a germ-food growth plate (agar plate) if a particular mold was also growing on the plate. Stated another way, when certain germs failed to grow in a germ-food growth plate it indicated that the plate was moldy.

This was an immensely important medical paradigm-shifting fact, another very big deal which also would eventually

change the world forever as did Jenner's medical blockbuster discovery about one hundred years earlier.

Fleming's mold was called Penicillium, a primitive organism which unknown to anyone before that time had developed in its DNA, a code to create a natural defense system that somehow killed other germs (gram positive staining bacteria). Penicillin and the antibiotic industry which it directly spawned has benefited humanity extraordinarily over decades. Penicillin's antibiotic activity came into existence under the profound influences of forces such as, natural selection and many other profound, complex, poorly understood, survival-based, gene pool affecting, naturally occurring evolutionary forces. In other words, Fleming did not invent an antibiotic; he found it. He found it hiding in nature.

That is what I believe the sincere Fleming was trying to explain at the Nobel after-party.

Almost certainly he was also trying to teach us something.

"I was only observing nature."

Perhaps he should have shouted, "NATURE holds the key to science!"

Yet, Fleming's comments embody a scientific notion of enduring value to the human race.

Here are Dr. Albert Einstein's comments on the very same topic:

"Look deeply into nature, and then you will understand everything,"

And, continues Dr. Einstein:

"We only know one thousandth of one percent of what nature has to teach us."

Nature, of course, includes the entire real universe, which is composed of scientifically proven and many still unproven realities, ranging in size and scope, starting from subatomic, to atomic, to molecular, to bio-molecular, to biological, to geophysical, to astrophysical to galactic and to intergalactic realities.

The natural human immune organ system reality and natural penicillin antibiotic activity reality discoveries changed the world forever once humanity became aware of them.

However, both processes had been occurring in nature since before our ancestors first stood up on their hind legs.

Man has done nothing to create or invent these natural phenomena.

They were discovered, not invented - a monumentally significant distinction.

Great advances in medicine are discovered in nature and not invented by man, although we benefit when we are wise enough to study nature intelligently to discover her great secrets.

Medical Paradigm Shifts
Medical paradigm shifts are rare.

The last two were unanticipated colossal steps explosively triggered by singularly critical yet remarkably simple observations of nature made by single persons who eventually challenged current day scientific medical thinking. Changes in medical thinking alter the focus of **medical scientific research,** which then and only then triggers the paradigm shift to begin its quantum leap in human benefits. It is the change in focus of medical research which actually triggers the benefits to society. That is what we need now.

From science to culture

An important medical observation is largely an individual's event, but disseminating the meaning of the new observation is a shared cultural event that must occur adequately if anyone is to benefit.

Medical history teaches us that these rare quantum leaps in medical practices cannot and will not happen unless and until the significance of the observation is properly disseminated. The new discovery and its implications must become known to a tipping point of significantly credible people by whatever means available within the culture.

Then another critical mass of consciousness about the discovery and its implications must reach a critical mass before the discovery can do anybody any good. And history teaches us that if the new quantum information is not adequately disseminated and communicated, it dies for an indefinite period of time measurable only in retrospect, until the observation is again made by someone connected to a more effective voice.

"All truth passes through three stages.

First, it is ridiculed.

Second, it is violently opposed.

Third, it is accepted as being self-evident."

(Arthur Schopenhauer)

Medical knowledge, especially great medical knowledge, does little good unless it is widely shared.

And there are formidable forces in play, which history teaches us will always serve to resist a new and higher level of medical consciousness within any culture. The news of an important medical observation must penetrate the cultural resistance to it. (I refer you to the concept of "memes," new ideas that propagate by certain likely pathways of communication as explained by the study of memetics.)

Example 1: The existence of the human immune system first penetrated the consciousness of a requisite critical mass of people around 1786 A.D., triggered by a simple observation of nature, an observable reality in milkmaids, which became the mother of the "immunity idea" (the immunity meme), an idea which once finally accepted and consciously understood by enough people triggered a paradigm shift in medical thinking, which changed the focus of attention in medical scientific research.

Example 2: The next big event happened about a hundred years later when a natural reality within a moldy culture dish was observed, fostering the "antibiotic idea" (the antibiotic meme). Once the new medical idea and its implications became accepted and consciously understood by enough people around 1899 A.D., the focus of medical research shifted. Research quickly developed inexpensive, reliable and safe penicillin antibiotics and an entire industry of derivative antibiotic inventions which are absolutely indispensable in medicine today. The amount of human suffering and premature death eliminated by antibiotics is incalculable. Other than vaccines, nothing even comes close in profundity in all of medical science, before or since, except for the huge medical notion called the "germ theory," which lead ulti-

Roger M. Nocera, M.D.

mately to public sanitation, medical sterilization, vaccines, and to antibiotics themselves.

CHAPTER TWO

A New Scientific Medical Discovery

"If we work on the assumption that what is accepted as
true, is really true,

there would be little hope for advance."

(Orville Wright)

Roger M. Nocera, M.D.

THE NEXT QUANTUM LEAP IN MEDICINE

In the first decade of this century, nearly 200 years after the discovery of the immune system and 100 years after the discovery of penicillin, the next big observation in medical science occurred, and like all the others it had been there all along, naturally, a part of nature, as if waiting to be observed.

Here and now in 2011 it is a bit difficult to pinpoint to whom the credit for this magnificent discovery should go. A number of individuals around the world have contributed. Rather than claim to be sure, I will leave it to the medical historians to decide the issue.

Since the critical medical observation of nature happened largely in the first decade of this century, between 2000 and 2010[1, 4], the responsible individuals can be called the Twenty-First Century, decade-one cell-scientists, or the 2000-DOCS.

Background. The following are undisputed medical scientific facts and in essence the sum total of what the worldwide medical establishment knew about stem cells as we entered the year 2000.

Stem cells make cells different from themselves.

- Most all cells make other cells.

- All cells are either non-stem cells or stem cells.

- Most cells are non-stem cells.

- Only stem cells can make cells that are different from themselves.

· Making a cell different from itself is what makes a stem cell a stem cell.

· Non-stem cells are cells that do not make cells different from themselves.

There are only two situations in normal unadulterated human biology where there are "cells that make cells different from themselves."

A human embryo starts off with one cell, a zygote, created by the union of a sperm and egg. By the end of pregnancy human babies have trillions of cells, but only 220 different types of cells. We are born with all 220 different cell types and they stay with us from cradle to grave. We call all these different cell types **"adult" cells**. The medical term "adult" as it refers to cells means the cells we are naturally born with. So the sometimes confusing reality is that babies when they are born, according to the scientific language conventions, have only adult cells in their bodies. We think of babies as being non-adults, and they are, of course, but science refers to cells as "adult" if and only if those cells are normally in the human baby at birth. There are heart adult cells, brain adult cells, liver adult cells, etc.

Simple logic demands that any process that starts with one cell type and ends with 220 different cell types must have cells "that make other cell types different from themselves." Specifically, **"embryonic stem cells,** which are found in the early embryo can produce all 220 different cell types found in humans. All the embryonic stem cells are used up normally long before a baby is born.

Adult stem cells
The second place in biology that we have known about stem cells (cells that make cells different from themselves) is in bone

marrow, where there are cells that throughout life make all the body's blood cells: red blood cells, all the various white blood cells, as well as platelets.

The cells that make blood cells are not themselves blood cells, so this is a circumstance in which one cell type makes a different cell type, so we call them "stem cells" too.

A red blood cell doesn't make another red blood cell; another type of cell, a stem cell produces them.

This is a process in which one cell type makes a different cell type, which defines a stem cell, and since these stem cells are post-natal, found after birth, they are called adult stem cells.

This is information about embryonic and adult stem cells we have known for many decades, and as I was taught in medical school over 30 years ago.

Before 2000 the world wide medical establishment believed, and many unfortunately still believe, that bone marrow adult stems have no other biological function than to exclusively make blood cells.

That belief is terribly incorrect, a huge and long standing error in humanity's medical perception of the actual reality of adult stem cells' normal, natural biological functions.[1,2]

"In the matter of a difficult question it is more
likely that the truth should have been discovered
by the few than by the many."

(Rene Descartes)

The New Discovery

In various experiments in lab animals the 2000-DOCS were able to label bone marrow cells and then put them into an animal that has had its bone marrow removed by radiation or chemotherapy (marrow ablated).

The new labeled bone marrow cells automatically make an entirely new full functioning bone marrow to replace the one that was removed from the lab animal (allogeneic transplantation and engraftment with marrow organ regeneration).[1]

Under this scientific model, whatever the labeled bone marrow cells did biologically could be followed and traced. These labels could be seen and identified when any tissue that contained them was viewed under a special microscope. Therefore, if one of the labeled adult stem cells of the new bone marrow turned into another type of cell, as stem cells do, the new cell type would have the tell-tale label when viewed under a high-power tissue microscope.

Of course, it wasn't long before the laboratory animals' blood cells started to be produced by labeled bone marrow adult stem cells. The labeled bone marrow adult stem cells were making new blood cells that had the labels (the old science).

Then they did something simple and brilliant, which is destined to change the world forever as momentously as vaccines and antibiotics.

So that these sacrificial animals' lives will not have been sacrificed in vain, please with reverence to the animals' collective potential contribution to mankind, please pay attention to the science, for which these animals gave their lives.

The lab animals were purposely given a severe injury to their hearts (induced myocardial infarctions by ligation of one of the coronary arteries).

After waiting for the rats to recover from their induced heart attacks (weeks), they examined their repaired heart tissue under a powerful microscope (histological cardiac section microscopy).

There were new normal heart cells that grew back in the injured animals' hearts, repairing it, and all of them bore the new bone marrow cell labels! [1]

The labeled bone marrow adult stem cells had to have found their way specifically to the injured part of the heart and then repaired it, by transforming into heart cells, as stem cells can do, to replace the dead heart cells. All the replacement heart cells had the labels, because they were coming from the labeled bone marrow cells, all of them.

Labeled heart cells were never put into the animals, only bone marrow adult stem cells.

The new bone marrow adult stem cells were healing the animal's heart by replacing the dead heart cells with new heart cells!

They wondered if this healing from the bone marrow adult stem cells also worked the same in brain injuries.

What if the same experiment was performed but instead of causing heart injury, the 2000-DOCS injured the animals' brains instead?

Would the bone marrow labeled adult stem cells be somehow naturally delivered from the bone marrow specifically to the injured brain site and transform into new brain cells to fix the brain tissue damage?

Would the labeled adult stem cells heal brain tissue too? So they then injured the animals' brains (an induced cerebral infarct by ligation of one of the rat's carotid arteries). After injuring their brains, they waited for them to recover. They then examined their brain tissue under a microscope.

Reality happens.

The microscopic exam of the recovered animals' brains showed repair and replacement of dead brain cells with new brain cells and all these new brain cells had the labels when viewed under the microscope.

These new labeled brain cells were no longer bone marrow adult stem cells because they had transformed themselves into new replacement brain cells, as they had done with replacement heart cells.

In both the heart and brain tissue, the cellular healing had to be due to adult stem cells of the labeled bone marrow adult stem cell pool because the original labels were not put on brain cells or heart cells but only on adult stem cells.

That is the discovery which is about to change our world.

Similar types of label marrow adult stem cell tracing experiments eventually demonstrated this tissue repair by bone marrow adult stem cells occurred in virtually every organ they tested, including the liver, pancreas, bone, skeletal muscle, spinal cord, thyroid, lungs, etc.

These experiments confirmed that bone marrow adult stem cells not only are making all the various blood cells, as we always believed, but also, adult bone marrow stem cells are also repairing any injury in the liver, kidneys, brain, heart, lungs, bone, etc., whenever they are damaged by disease or injury[1,2].

For the first time in history there was proof of a natural **healing organ system** composed of bone marrow adult stem cells that were long believed, almost religiously by our world's medical experts, to only be making blood cells. Of course, now it had to proven unequivocally that the same thing happened in humans and not just in rats - but they could hardly purposely injure the human patients' hearts and brains to see if their bone marrow would send out labeled cells to heal them.

Bone marrow transplant patients

Leukemia is treated with radiation and chemotherapy. But along with the cancer cells these harsh treatments also destroy bone marrow cells, all of them. This is called bone marrow ablation, a side effect of such treatments.

Without bone marrow the cancer patients will die, so a new bone marrow is transplanted in order to rescue such patients from a certain death after the cancer is killed by the chemotherapy and radiation therapy. If the bone marrow donor is male and the recipient of the new bone marrow is female, then the Y-chromosome can be used as a label under a microscope, simply by using a special Y-chromosome microscopic stain.

Females effectively only have XX-chromosomes in their native body tissues. If a female cancer patient receives a bone marrow transplant from a male donor, we have a serendipitous adult stem cell label, just like the laboratory animal experiment. Effectively, the new male bone marrow in a female recipient patient is labeled by the Y-chromosome.

Postmortem tissue examination of female bone marrow transplant patients who had years earlier received a male donor bone marrow revealed many Y-chromosome cells throughout their bodies, which would only be present if they came from the donated male bone marrow adult stem cells. There were brain cells, liver cells, heart cells and more, all created by adult stem cells that gave them each and all Y-chromosomes. Over many years these cancer survivors would suffer from cell damage in various parts of their bodies from a variety of ailments before they died.

Obviously whenever these patients would get sick or injured the labeled bone marrow adult stem cells would be sent out from the donated male bone marrow to somehow locate the injury and heal the problem by making new cells to replace the dead ones, wherever the cell damage was located in the body[2]. The staining Y-chromosomes were found in vastly greater numbers in the liver if the patient had liver disease between the time of her bone marrow transplant and death.

A vocabulary change

"A word is not unchanged; it is the skin of a living thought and may vary greatly according to the circumstances and the time in which it is used."

(Oliver Wendell Holmes)

As you can see "adult stem cells" were not newly discovered. We have known about adult stem cells that make blood cells in bone marrow for decades. Therefore the meaning of the phrase "adult stem cells" has been changing in complex medically important ways as we have been learning the biological activities and potential medical activities that they actually have.

The phrase simply does not mean what it used to mean and is, therefore, now treacherous to engage for both readers and writers, both listeners and speakers. Since many of the exact same adult stem cells (phenotypes) that make blood cells are also the same ones found to be healing the body too, one cannot say that "adult stem cells" were the new discovery. Therefore, the term "adult stem cells" should be avoided as much as possible, especially for non-scientists, because it has been contaminated with a Tower of Babel-like character in the public's mind which obscures the truth of the new medical discovery.

So what is the new discovery exactly, precisely, if it was not "adult stem cells"?

The discovery was literally that some cells, adult stem cells found in our human bone marrow, heal the body naturally and continuously throughout our lives... (ergo the title of this book, Cells That Heal Us From Cradle To Grave, A Quantum Leap in Medical Science))

I refer to the new science as "Healing Cells" instead of adult stem cells. I'm not trying to give the topic a snappy, marketable name. I use the vocabulary "Healing Cells" so that the wording sheds light, instead of confusion, on the public's consciousness of this extraordinary and timely medical discovery.

"If language is not correct, then what is said is not what

is meant;

Hence there must be no arbitrariness in what is said.

This matters above everything."

(Confucius)

These Healing Cells have their home base of operation within human bone marrow. The genetic code for this healing system is imbedded within our DNA, of course.

Healing Cells are the body's method of healing itself and this human healing organ system works constantly throughout our lives, just like our hearts beat without stopping until we die and just as our immune organ system sends out cells (phagocytes) that kill invaders (micro-pathogens) and cancer throughout our lives. This is all now scientific fact, whether it is acknowledged or not.

There is nothing that medical science or doctors have done to cause this natural cellular healing organ system. Indeed, all this has been going on naturally just as natural immunity and natural penicillin antibiotic activity had since before our ancestors first stood up on their hind legs.

Starting a new medical biotech company

"Prayer indeed is good, but while calling on the gods a man should himself lend a hand."

(Hippocrates)

A few of us doctors believed that it was critically and historically profound that certain human adult stem cells were playing a major biological role in a previously unrecognized **human cellular healing organ system.** Compelled by this historic discovery, a few of us got together to form a new medical international biotechnology organization to begin the hard work of developing this new medical science clinically. Here is why we believed in our medical cause:

It was the human immune organ system that Dr. Edward Jenner discovered which had such profound, unprecedented and lasting benefit to our world, which we still enjoy and depend on today. An organ system is biologically complex and integrated at multiple levels with all other human body organ systems. Any and all organ system failures can kill a patient; therefore, organ systems are medically very important to every physician and every patient.

There are volumes of important medical information to know about every organ system, so medical science is carved up into specialties based upon them, such as gastroenterology, obstetrics, cardiology, pulmonology, neurology and endocrinology.

It wasn't just any organ system that was discovered; it was "a human healing organ system," so it is particularly important to medicine.

We now know there are Healing Cells that compose a human bone marrow-based healing organ system, which is every bit as natural, complex and important to us medically as the human immune organ system, the cardiovascular organ system, the gastro-intestinal organ system, and the central nervous organ system.

Can you imagine medical doctors and medical scientists not being aware of any one of those basic biological human body organ systems?

Yet, before the first decade of this century no natural human healing organ system or bone marrow-based natural healing cells were demonstrated to exist nor widely believed to exist by the vast worldwide professional medical establishment.

Why do we get sick?

All diseases make us sick by injuring or killing body cells. So why don't Healing Cells heal all wounds and diseases if they already occur naturally within our bodies?

It has now been scientifically established that there often comes a point when diseases or injuries require many more Healing Cells than our bodies can produce in time. It has also been well documented that aging and the effects of disease can and often do overwhelm the ability of our Healing Cells to heal us, in ways we can scientifically measure now.

This is where medical therapy can come in. Imagine if doctors focused their treatments on supplying the required number and type of healthy Healing Cells to the site of disease or injury. If we can replace injured body cells with Healing Cells, how could improvements in health and healing not follow?

Is there any medical problem that could not be reversed and improved if our bodies received adequate doses of just the right type and amount of Healing Cells at the correct intervals when we get sick?

At this point in our experience and medical research, the answer appears to be a resounding no.

Most people, both in and out of medicine, still do not understand the vast quantum leap in medical science that this discovery represents. Yet something great and wonderful has happened that could be very helpful and very close at hand, as humanity struggles to navigate beyond a rough first decade of the Twenty-First Century.

A true story

Although I shared the experience of the physician with heart disease earlier please allow me to give the full account of the case here, to document the details more fully. Many more examples of treatment successes are found later in this book.

The middle-aged man was suffering from a very serious heart disease that ran in his family. He already had to watch helplessly as two of his beloved family members including his mother died painfully of the same fatal heart disease that was now killing him.

He was himself a medical doctor, so he had an exquisitely sensitive perspective on just how grave his medical condition actually was. In fact, the poor doctor was using an accurate and sophisticated medical laboratory test called the "cardiac ejection fraction" to gruesomely inform himself exactly how long he had left to live.

The doctor's heart ejection fraction is the percentage of the blood inside his heart that it can pump out with every heartbeat. The ill doctor knew all too well that patients with his heart disease invariably experience a decline in their heart's ejection fraction as they approach a painful death.

A normal ejection fraction is about 55 percent, and by the time it declines to a weakened 10 percent, death soon follows as the patient slowly drowns in his own heart-failure lung fluid (pulmonary edema from chronic progressive congestive heart failure).

The doctor's heart ejection fraction had already dwindled down to a terrifying 30 percent when he contacted me in what I can only describe as a state of reserved panic. With a cardiac ejection fraction of only 30 percent he was half way to the end, and he knew it.

To make matters worse he had spent all his money and savings for medical expenses and burial costs for his family's fatal illnesses and he had long since been unable to practice medicine following his own ill heart's downward trajectory into failure.

According to his personal team of doctors he would soon be dead if he didn't get a heart transplant, which he rightfully dreaded because he knew it would be very painful, extremely physically invasive and dangerous, and would cost a quarter of a million dollars—that is if he could raise the necessary funds and a suitable heart could be found for him before he died.

Can you imagine how alone, defeated, frightened and sick this man must have felt?

In October 2005 this desperately ill doctor contacted me in my official capacity as chief medical officer for our newly formed adult stem cell international biotechnology company. He asked me if I would use whatever influence I had to help get him accepted as a patient in one of our company's affiliate Central American clinics. Of course, he had no money, and as in all new clinics, ours relied on patient fees to financially survive and to be able to serve and help the next sick patient.

At this time (2005), our entire medical advisory board and I doubted that our cell treatment therapy would actually help the good doctor. So we had to decide whether to treat this ill man despite our therapeutic efficacy doubts and the unreimbursed costs to the new company.

In the end our scholarly therapeutic medical analysis meant nearly nothing, as the doctor's profound suffering had hijacked our collective sense of compassion, and we decided to help him if we could.

Although we had reservations about the outcome, we were comforted by the fact that the treatment would not harm the doctor (now patient) in any way, because it never harms anyone. We knew that after giving him the cell treatment the worst that could happen was nothing, which in the doctor's case would be terrible enough. We knew that the high quality medical methods of these professionally performed transplantations of cells would not hurt the doctor nor diminish his hope of receiving a heart transplant if one became available – as small as that hope was.

Through a little arm vein we injected the gravely ill doctor with healthy, live Healing Cells, which were obtained from a healthy afterbirth following a normal full-term delivery. (In this book, parenthesized information is especially for the doctors; not reading them will not lessen your grasp of the all-important big picture. The technical verbiage for our treatment of the doctor was an allogeneic transplantation of cytokine-triggered cell-culture expansion progeny of isolated human afterbirth derived— CD 34 positive and mesenchymal adult stem cell phenotypes.

The doctor was given these healing cells and it required no drugs for immune suppression, as it never does in our hands.

We were shocked
Shortly after the treatment the doctor started to feel better and regained much of his energy. A few months after receiving these natural Healing Cells the doctor's heart ejection fraction started to go up instead of continuing its progressive downward trend.

That result was beyond our expectations—beyond our hope! We felt that a success in this case would be getting him another year of life plus some hope for future advances.

To our delight and surprise four months after this simple, painless Healing Cell treatment, the previously gravely ill doctor **had recovered completely**. Most will not recognize the incredible importance of this statement, but all medical professionals will understand the unprecedented success of this procedure and the sublime implications for the future of medicine. As one of my non-medical friends put it: "We have just arrived at the age of Star Trek medicine."

Patient follow up: The doctor has now withdrawn from all heart failure medications, has normal blood heart enzyme profiles, has a normal cardiac ejection fraction of 55 percent, and is back practicing medicine and exercising vigorously. He is healthier than I am! We have since successfully treated many patients for heart disease, often with similar history-making, documented success.[25]

Roger M. Nocera, M.D.

CHAPTER THREE

Measuring Healing Cells in Blood

"Old age is no place for sissies."

(Bette Davis)

How Healing Cells Work

All diseases hurt us by injuring and killing our cells. When cells die they leak out biochemically powerful substances called cytokines, which accumulate in two places; first at the site of tissue injury and then eventually the cytokines spill over into the blood, circulating with it throughout the body. We can measure the various cytokine blood levels. The cytokines stimulate the bone marrow healing organ system to make more adult stem cells and we can measure a rise in the adult stem cell blood count shortly after a rise in blood cytokine levels are measureable.

Cytokines, by a well-documented process called chemoattraction, literally trigger the movement of adult healing stem cells to move toward the injury site concentrating them around the **injury so they can produce replacement cells to repair the tissue damage** by another well documented process called cellular transdifferentiation. (see addendum for details and insight into these fascinating biological processes)

> "The art of medicine consists in amusing the patient while nature cures the disease."
>
> (Voltaire)

Just like a white blood cell count, we can now measure a sick patient's Healing Cells blood count.

Moreover, just as a white blood cell count is a way to measure a patient's ability to mount a good cell defense against infection, a Healing Cells blood count is a way to measure a patient's ability to mount a good Healing Cells defense against tissue injury from disease.

Infections (and other disease attacks) that are trivial to young, healthy patients can and often do kill older and otherwise sicker patients. This is not a new medical idea; rather it is quite medically fundamental, likely dating back to Hippocrates.

Older and sick patients often die of lung infections (pneumonia), many of which occur when old and sick patients are in the hospital with their oldness and sickness (nosocomial opportunistic pneumonitis). Their immune systems can't make enough healthy, well-functioning white blood cells fast enough to fight off the invasion of some germ (bacterial inoculate) in order to recover from the lung infection. This is essentially a fight between the patient's white blood cells and the germs.

It is accepted medical fact that an elevated white blood count is expected in young patients with infections, like appendicitis and pneumonia, but this is not necessarily true of an elderly and sickly patient because their white blood cell counts often do not rise as they should because their bone marrow is worn down with age and disease. No well-trained physician would hesitate to diagnose appendicitis or pneumonia if suspected in an elderly patient just because the patient does not have the usual elevated white blood cell count seen routinely in younger patients who get these diseases also.

So the elderly patient dies of infections that a younger and healthier patient would not. More precisely, the infection would never beat the army of white blood cells that young patients can produce and deliver in time to prevent the germs from getting the upper hand.

We see the same thing when doctors are forced to give drugs to suppress the immune system, which causes the same problem of getting hurt by otherwise minor infectious germs (opportunistic infections). Therefore, as you can see this idea of human cell systems failing under pressure from disease and age is not new. Now we find the same rules have been proven to apply to Healing Cells, and why not it is the same bone marrow that produces white blood cells and Healing Cells.

It has recently been discovered that after a stroke, which is the rapid death of brain cells, there is a measurable rise in bone marrow Healing Cells production (CD34+cells) and release of these cells into the blood, raising their numbers in the blood, which we can also measure (CD34+ adult stem cell blood count).

We can now effectively predict the clinical outcome of a stroke by measuring the Healing Cell blood count.

If a high enough Healing Cells blood count (CD34+ adult stem cell blood count) has not been achieved by one month after any stroke, we can now use that objective information to predict that the patient will not recover from the stroke neurologically, whereas if the Healing Cells blood count (CD34+cell blood count) is higher than a certain value at one month after a stroke, then the patient's neurological recovery can be accurately predicted. This has now been proven.[10]

Despite these new discoveries, can you believe there are no clinical studies in our country whereby stroke patients are given their own Healing Cells, CD34 + cells, or better, afterbirth-derived, physiologically robust and perfectly safe Healing Cells (allogeneic cord blood CD34 + expansion progeny) for a month after their strokes?

Stroke patients often live for years as invalids, draining family and government financial recourses to pay for their many hospitalizations, until the physical inactivity caused by their stroke degrades their health and they die.

Although now proven scientifically, this critically revealing new information has not been well disseminated to our doctors, and they remain relatively, if not completely unconscious of these newly established medical facts about stem cells. Doctors do not know that they can measure their stroke patients' Healing Cells blood count (CD34+cell blood count) to predict their recovery or lack of recovery from a stroke. They do not know enough to be outraged that they are forbidden to help their stroke patients by prescribing the many safe ways there are to give such patients help with supplemental Healing Cells (phenotype CD+34). Yes, Healing Cells treatment will actually change the outcome of the stroke rather than just measure the resulting damage.

Our artery disease epidemic

The disease that kills more Americans annually than all other diseases combined, including all cancers, is called hardening of the arteries, or atherosclerosis (ath-er-o-skleh-RO-sis), a condition in which fatty material collects along the walls of arteries. The fatty material thickens, hardens (forms calcium deposits), and may eventually block the arteries when clotted. Hardening of the arteries (atherosclerosis) is the cause of most heart disease, strokes and serious leg circulation problems (claudication of atherosclerotic peripheral vascular disease, PVD and limb ischemia).

The first and only sign or symptom of this disease for about 250,000 Americans yearly is sudden death. Many do not understand that the sophisticated exercise image-assisted **cardiac stress test** can be entirely normal on Thursday and a deadly heart attack can happen on Friday. This is a sneaky disease when it involves the arteries that supply the heart.

A patient needs at least a 60 percent narrowing of one of the heart arteries to have an abnormal stress test, yet, the majority of heart attacks, even the fatal ones, happen because of sudden artery thrombosis in heart arteries that are far less than the 60 percent required for an abnormal stress test.

Hardening of the arteries (atherosclerosis) is a disease of the arteries' lining cells (an endothelial cell disease). The first event in the causation (pathogenesis) of all hardening of the arteries is injury to the inner lining cells of the arteries (endothelial cells).

Whenever the inner lining cells of arteries are exposed to unfriendly internal conditions such as high blood cholesterol or high blood pressure or smoke toxins, etc., there is resultant injury to the inner lining cells of the arteries, some of which die and spill their cytokine substances into the neighboring tissues and into the blood.

The elevated blood cytokine substance level hormonally stimulates bone marrow tissue to produce and release cells certain adult stem cells called endothelial precursor-Healing Cells[10, 11, 12] (EPCs), which because of cytokine chemo-attraction effects accumulate at the site of the injured arterial inner wall lining cells' tissue neighborhood.

The cytokines influence the Healing Cells (EPCs) to transform (cellular trans-differentiate) into inner lining artery cells (endothelial cells) to replace the injured artery lining cells that were damaged.

This cellular process goes on as needed continuously and endlessly, unless and until the part of the Healing Cells organ system responsible for arterial wall repair wears out from exhaustion and endothelial precursor-Healing Cells depletion over the years.

In other words, we use up all of those artery inner lining precursor-Healing Cells or the ability to produce them and the system breaks down from wear and tear.

It has now been established that just as we measure a patient's white blood cell count to see if a patient has an infection, we can likewise measure a patient's inner artery lining precursor-Healing Cells count (EPC blood count) to accurately predict if the patient has significant artery narrowing from atherosclerosis or not! [10, 11, 12]

Once hardening of the arteries takes hold, the Healing Cells blood count goes down, because the disease has finally gotten the upper hand on the Healing Cells system, and this suppresses it, just like too much work for too long wears out the white blood cell-making capacity of other parts of the bone marrow in old patients with pneumonia.

We measure how much artery narrowing disease a patient has in the heart by a test, a heart artery picture-gram (coronary arteriogram). We can now predict the outcome of such a test just by measuring the patient's Healing Cells blood count (Endothelial Precursor Cells, EPC blood count). If a patient can maintain this particular type of Healing Cells blood count (EPC blood count) above a certain number we can predict that the patient's arteries will be normal when we do this sophisticated test. This is true because a high Healing Cells blood count is proof that a patient's Healing Cells system is keeping up with the demand for inner artery lining cell replacement and will not have atherosclerosis. But if a patient's Healing Cells blood count (Endothelial Precursor Cells, EPCs) is lower than a certain number range, we can predict with confidence that the patient's natural healing stem cell system has been defeated by the artery hardening disease process.

Only after the Healing Cells organ system has been over-whelmed, a measurable event, by the constant need to re-place dying arterial wall lining cells will a patient begin to develop the characteristic artery narrowing disease responsi-ble for most deaths in America.

It's easy to see that safe supplemental injections of Healing Cells (specifically EPCs) would save lives and eliminate much human suffering if doctors were allowed to give these cells in the many safe ways we now know to give them to help our patients.

Naturally transplanted Healing Cells

Autologous Healing Cells (auto=your own) by definition come from the same patient receiving them for treatment, whereas, allogeneic Healing Cells (allo=from elsewhere) come from a source other than the patient receiving them.

Let's imagine that we take some of your Healing Cells out of your blood (leukophoresis) and put them into a syringe ready for injection.

If we inject them back into your body we will have performed an **autologous transplantation**, from you to you, and we call the cells we injected into you autologous Healing Cells.

But if those same cells are instead injected into me, we will have performed an **allogeneic transplantation,** and those same cells must now be referred to as allogeneic.

As unapparent as it might seem, the idea to supplement a per-son's Healing Cells organ system with Healing Cells from some-one else (allogeneic cell transplantation) is not an original idea. This idea was plagiarized directly from the original author . . . nature itself.

It has recently been scientifically proven that every mother during pregnancy receives a Healing Cells transplantation from each of her babies, an ubiquitous natural allogeneic transplantation called human maternal microchimerism.

For instance, we have found that all mothers have their babies' Healing Cells within their bone marrow. All mothers have within their body tissues cells that were transplanted and turned into other cell types (trans-differentiated) from each of their babies when these cells passed through the placenta from baby's blood to mother's blood. This natural transfer of cells from one person to another (allogeneic transplantation) occurs with every pregnancy.

Moreover, it has been recently shown that women live an average of an extra year longer for each three babies they give birth to, up to 14 children.[14]

It has been postulated that this increased life expectancy is due to the benefits of these (allogeneic) Healing Cells transplantations, which each and every mother receives from each and every one of her babies during each of her pregnancies.

In other words, unless she has passed on, your mother still has Healing Cells in her bone marrow donated from you. Also, she would have your donated cells functioning normally within her brain, liver, and heart, and all other tissues of her body. Furthermore, if a mother gets sick during or even after her pregnancy, her baby's Healing Cells will help to heal her because of this very natural process encoded in our human DNA, whereby baby's cells are found living in every mother's body (maternal microchimerism).

Let's say a pregnant woman suffers from liver infection (hepatitis) in her late pregnancy (third trimester). The infection will cause damage to her liver cells, which in turn will spill their cytokine substances into the surrounding liver tissue neighborhood and into the blood. The rising blood cytokine levels will trigger the mother's bone marrow to produce and release Healing Cells, which will accumulate at the site of injury due to the chemoattraction effects of the increased liver tissue cytokine concentration.

But because all babies transfer many of their Healing Cells through the placenta into the mother's blood, the baby's Healing Cells also have an opportunity to respond to the cytokine chemoattraction within the mother's injured tissues, and they too will be attracted, accumulating within and repairing the mother's injured liver.[15] The baby's Healing Cells then respond to the biochemical hormonal signals of the cytokines in the maternal liver, which will cause them to transform (trans-differentiate) into new liver cells to replace the mother's injured and dying liver cells.

The baby's Healing Cells transform into liver cells that will stay with the mother for life, functioning normally to detoxify the mother's body as liver cells do. These are stunning scientific facts, newly discovered (maternal microchimerism).

This addition of the baby's cells into the mother's tissues is called maternal microchimerism, which is the result of nature's (allogeneic) Healing Cells transplantation. There is work being done on a way to perform genetic counseling to pregnant women, at Tufts Medical School, not by the somewhat dangerous baby cell retrieval method called amniocentesis, in which a long needle is stuck into the mothers abdominal wall, piercing the uterus to collect some of the baby cells floating in the fluid, which surrounds the baby during pregnancy. This procedure is invasive, painful and dangerous to mother and child.

Now there is work being done to retrieve baby cells for genetic counseling not by an invasive amniocentesis needle method, but rather, the baby's cells are obtained by drawing blood only from the mother,[14] knowing that the baby's Healing Cells have transplanted naturally there and are therefore in the mother's blood available to obtain and examine genetically via a simple blood draw with a tiny needle into the mother's arm vein.

You must admit, this is amazing new science.

It should be noted that you will find very few physicians that are educated and conscious that all mothers receive cells from all their babies which stay with them for life (maternal microchimerism), yet it is an immensely important and illustrious element of the Healing Cells organ system discovery.

Importantly, baby Healing Cells are much more robust and powerful than Healing Cells found within an older person.[17, 18, 19, 20, 21, 22, 23] This should be no surprise since babies are known to have amazing healing capacity; just ask any pediatrician or pediatric surgeon.

Baby Healing Cells duplicate exponentially faster than older people's Healing Cells and they produce exponentially more of those important hormonally active cytokine substances which are critically important because of their healing effects (trophic effects).

This is why baby afterbirth, the umbilical cords and placentas are so valuable to the human race. All babies leave a little of their blood behind within their afterbirth. That blood is rich in the baby's Healing Cells. We can extract these valuable robust Healing Cells from the afterbirth of normal deliveries and expand them into millions of usable therapeutic cells, which can be given to anyone, any patient for help with a disease.

Some cells age more than others

Because Healing Cells contain a very special substance called "telomerase," when they reproduce they don't age in the process.

DNA is a very long molecule. DNA loses some of its length (telomere DNA shortening) whenever the cell reproduces. This special substance (telomerase) prevents DNA shortening during reproduction of the cells that contain it.

Normal body (somatic) cells do not have this special substance (telomerase); therefore, their DNA gets shorter with every reproduction cycle. Once their DNA gets to a critical shortened length the cells die (apoptosis).

This cell reproduction limit (the Hayflick cellular reproduction limit[36]) is one of the reasons human beings age. Over time the shortening of our body cells' DNA that occurs with each reproduction cycle eventually kills the cells.

Because Healing Cells have this special substance (telomerase) within them they can reproduce over and over without the aging effects of shortened DNA.[24]

Therefore, Healing Cells can be duplicated (expanded in number) by stimulating them with cytokines in cell cultures, which causes them to exponentially duplicate into enormous numbers without aging, because they don't suffer from the DNA shortening reproduction limitations of somatic cells due to the special power of natural telomerase.

Let's look at a similar phenomenon to aid in our understanding of this critical concept.

In the days before digital media, offices revolved around the photocopier. Indeed, before that, there was carbon paper. If you didn't wish to type the same document more than once, you would place a sheet of carbon paper behind the surface sheet of paper you intended to type on, and then would place a sheet of paper behind the carbon paper. When the typewriter type-bar struck the letter imprinted on it against the ink ribbon, it would imprint the letter in ink on the sheet of paper. The impact would also cause a copy to be made on the second sheet of paper through the same process—the same outline of the letter would pass through the ink ribbon, the sheet of paper, and the carbon paper, leaving a similar impression on the second sheet of paper. However, the imprint on the second sheet would not be as sharp as the original, having lost quality and clarity due to the intervening sheet of paper and carbon paper. If you wished to make two or three copies at the same time, you needed only to stack more sheets of alternating carbon paper and white paper behind the original. Of course, with each successive copy, the clarity and quality would be reduced until by several copies deep, you couldn't read the printing very well.

When photocopiers came along, secretaries leaped with joy, because you could make an unlimited number of copies from the original, and each would be as clear as the last—although none would be quite as clear as the original. However, if you didn't have the original and needed to make a copy of one of the copies, that Third Generation copy would begin to show noticeable signs of quality and clarity loss. A copy of a Third Generation copy would render a Fourth Generation copy, and a copy of that would render a Fifth Generation copy. At some point in making generational copies, there is not enough clarity and quality to render a usable copy.

It is much like this in the regeneration of cells in our bodies.

Most of our regular (somatic) body cells are the type that contains little or no telomerase. So when such a cell is replaced, it is substituted with a Second Generation cell with shortened DNA. When that cell is replaced it is substituted with a Third Generation cell, and so on.

When I was young I once heard someone say that all of the cells in our body are replaced every seven years. Hallelujah! I thought, until I learned that each cell substitution was made with a cheap knockoff of the prior generation, which was a cheap knockoff of its prior generation, and so on.

Indeed, this is a very important process in aging. Our skin, muscles and organs all get older because the cells continually lose some of their original quality and clarity. DNA is damaged not only by a huge list of toxins each cell is exposed to over the years, but also by the cost of reproduction, DNA shortening (DNA telomere loss).

At some point, some of the cells fail to do their job altogether, leading to accelerated cell death. When total cell death exceeds total new cell replacement the aging process accelerates further—eventually and inevitably as the totality of cellular function fails beyond some multifactorial critical tipping point the entire unit shuts down . . . and we die.

The exciting news about Healing Cells is that they contain enough of this special substance (telomerase) to not have to suffer generational loss when they reproduce.

Therefore, we can stimulate Healing Cells to reproduce over and over again without losing their quality or originality. Can you see the implications of this extraordinary phenomenon?

Yes, we have arrived at the point where we can repair damaged tissues with cells that do not age the same way as other body cells do when they reproduce. We can duplicate these cells over and over in cell cultures after taking some of them out of a patient, giving us exponentially more Healing Cells to administer back into the patient. These cells go to work doing their natural healing activities, but in far greater numbers than the patient's body can produce in time without special help.

This very special substance (telomerase) found in Healing Cells adds to the staggering therapeutic potential of these cells when they are in capable clinical hands.

Recipients don't reject donated Healing Cells

Some might wonder how we can inject foreign Healing Cells from an unrelated baby's afterbirth into a stranger's body without getting rejection of the foreign cells by the patient's immune system given that we never administer immunosuppressive drugs.

This is yet another very exciting aspect of natural Healing Cells treatments.

As you probably know, whenever an organ is donated (a heart or kidney allogeneic organ transplant) in most cases the recipient's body will view the foreign organ as an attacking entity, and will retaliate to kill the invading tissue (transplant rejection). That is why patients must be given dangerous immune suppressing drugs after organ transplantation (especially if somewhat HLA antigen mismatched).

These drugs partly turn off the patient's immune system.

All babies' cells have genes that are half foreign (allogeneic) to its mother's genes because half of the baby's genes come from the father who, of course, is genetically unrelated to the mother.

As we now know, all babies successfully seed their mother's tissues with their Healing Cells (maternal microchimerism), which could only occur if there is something about baby Healing Cells that protects them from immune attack. Therefore, there must be a type of immune privilege by which baby Healing Cells are protected from immune attack from a foreign immune system (the mother's allogeneic immune system).

Moreover, the near universality of human maternal microchimerism is proof positive that there is immune privilege of all babies' Healing Cells because if there was no such intrinsic protection, the baby's cells would be killed by the mother's immune system, in which case mothers would never have their babies' cells living and functioning happily in mothers' bodies, which we know they actually do (the fact of universal maternal microchimerism).

This immune privilege, proven to exist by baby's Healing Cells unmolested involvement in mother's body (maternal microchimerism), is why we have not had to give immune suppressive drugs to our allogeneic Healing Cells therapy patients overseas.

All babies' Healing Cells are transplantable into foreign (allogeneic) immune system environments because that has been an integral part of their natural life cycle through our human evolutionary timeline. Babies' Healing Cells help to heal the mothers' bodies during and after each pregnancy, an enormous evolutionary survival advantage, which naturally selects for survival of those babies who make Healing Cells that can evade immune attack by their mothers' foreign immune systems. The survival advantage of mothers is likewise linked to those who have immune systems which do not attack their baby's Healing Cells.

The genes allowing this mutual symbiotic help from baby to mother to baby are selected for continuation within the gene pool naturally because such genes create survival advantage, whereas genes that do not provide for this symbiosis (maternal microchimerism) cannot get passed on to the next generation because of the intrinsic survival disadvantages of such genes.

We know maternal microchimerism is a universal trait in humans at this point in our evolutionary development, which is why I view the existence of human maternal microchimerism as a full throated and elegant endorsement by nature itself for the therapeutic value of allogeneic Healing Cells transplantation.

Moreover, if healing adult stem cells did not significantly heal the body, they would present no survival advantage, and their allogeneic nature (half DNA is paternal) would not be tolerated as it is not tolerated anywhere else in human biology. But simple Darwinian science explains maternal microchimerism of adult stem cell immune privilege in allogeneic maternal environments, but only if they heal well enough to have produced survival advantage.

All afterbirth Healing Cells are allogeneic when used for therapy and are much more robust and potent than older patient's own Healing Cells. Despite this extremely important truth about allogeneic afterbirth derived Healing Cells superior potency and immune safety, there is no scientific research being conducted in the U.S. with these allogeneic Healing Cells.

You must admit, this seems a bit strange, doesn't it?

Results

Let's review a few typical medical cases from our affiliate overseas clinics where the doctors administer both autologous and allogeneic Healing Cells to help their patients with various diseases.

Autism

A nine-year-old girl came to the overseas clinic because of autism. This little girl was so profoundly autistic that she had never uttered an intelligible word, not even to her siblings and parents. She could only grunt.

She was also typically autistic in her non-social and avoidance behavior. Autism is a disease in which there is medical controversy as to its cause. What is clear is that these children have temporal lobe brain damage, killed brain cells from decreased blood flow in their temporal lobes.

Within four months after multiple intravenous injections with Healing Cells into this little girl's arm vein, taken safely from the afterbirth of a normal pregnancy, she started to speak spontaneously. Her speech and other skills advanced so rapidly that she has since skipped grades at school and now gets along much better with her family and friends.

This child and her family have been changed profoundly for the better due to nature's Healing Cells that normally would have been thrown away in the bio-trash.

Many other autistic children have obtained similar, documented history-making results at our clinic.

One successfully treated autistic ten-year-old boy put it best upon experiencing improved ability to function normally in ways that were new to him when he said, "Hey Mom, I'm cool now!"

Spinal cord damage

A young man came to the clinic with his beautiful young bride and his mom and dad, for Healing Cells treatments. He had suffered spinal cord damage sustained in an automobile accident. This young man was devastated because he could not feel nor move from his mid chest downward; he was paralyzed from his spinal cord injury.

He was given multiple (allogeneic) Healing Cells injections into an arm vein and safely into his spinal canal (intrathecal) in addition to simultaneous physical therapy.

Following months of treatment this man is now virtually walking with assistance and has regained many of his neurological lower body functions, a therapeutic feat never obtained with any other known therapy.

Many other spinal cord damaged patients are being helped with healing cells in the few small maverick clinics that exist around the world.

Muscular dystrophy

We also had a child with Duchene's muscular dystrophy (one of "Jerry's kids") who could hardly lift his hands two inches from his side.

Within months after injecting his muscles with afterbirth derived Healing Cells he could raise his hands over his head and his muscles had grown considerably in size.

After treatment his muscle biopsy demonstrated the normal production of dystrophin, a substance never seen in Duchene's muscular dystrophy patient's muscles. Of course his pre-treatment muscle biopsy showed no dystrophin.

We have treated four patients with Muscular Dystrophy who have all improved clinically.

Cerebral Palsy

We have successfully treated many children with cerebral palsy with Healing Cells, which we obtain harmlessly from normal afterbirth.

While it remains clear that severe brain damage cannot be entirely reversed as yet, we were able to give many of these children enough neurological improvement with Healing Cells to function better, which often produces profound improvement in the quality of their daily lives and the lives of their caregivers.

For example, children with cerebral palsy that are unable to walk or feed themselves, while generally unable to become ambulatory with treatments at the current level of the technology, can often learn to feed themselves after receiving Healing Cells. This is a small but profoundly impactful change in their neurological status, and subsequently in the quality of their daily lives.

Most of the many cerebral palsy patients that we have treated do show significant life-altering neurological improvement after treatment.

Further improvement will undoubtedly be obtainable once we learn more about which cellular protocol parameters work best in these children and when we learn the many ways these healing effects can be augmented.

This is why we need more doctors involved in establishing treatment regimens and protocols, and why we need a national database in which we can accumulate all of this useful information and make it available to all treating physicians in America.

Rheumatoid arthritis and multiple sclerosis

Patients with rheumatoid arthritis are also helped, often dramatically with Healing Cells injections.

For these patients as well as those with other autoimmune diseases, we have discovered by simple trial and error that fat derived (autologous) Healing Cells from the patient's own body fat work best so far.

Healing Cells get trapped within fat tissue throughout our lives and are unable to escape from fat tissue into the blood in order to heal the body when needed. By simply removing some of the patient's fat tissue with liposuction and then "melting" the fat with a connective tissue dissolving enzyme (collagenase) we are able to release the Healing Cells from the fat within a test tube.

Once the patient's own Healing Cells are harvested in this way from liposuction fluid we are then able to re-inject just the Healing Cells back into the same patient's blood, which allows the previously "fat trapped" Healing Cells to travel throughout the blood to heal all injured tissues. **The treatment consists of releasing a patient's own fat-trapped Healing Cells so the cells are free to do what natural Healing Cells do . . . heal.**

We have gotten very good at treating MS and RA in our Central American clinics with the patient's own healing cells.

We have shown a high percentage of treatment results for both diseases now that we have found the best protocol so far.

Heart disease
After sharing the story of our first heart patient, I am quite pleased to further report that we have since treated many other patients with congestive heart failure problems with Healing Cells with similar medical history making success.

Trapped for life in fat
Healing Cells behave just like our immune organ system. Their work is never done, from cradle to grave, like our hearts, brains,

lungs, etc. There are always a few hundred thousand cells to re-place on a slow day. So, like a white blood cell count there is a base line range.

But if it's a busy day because the body is actively ill with an in-fection, trauma, environmental challenge or stress, then the Heal-ing Cells blood count goes way up, out of the statistically deter-mined "normal range." Just like a high white blood cell count happens with infection and is measurable, so too is an elevated Healing Cells blood count when the patient is fighting with any disease.

So imagine, all our lives, whenever we get the sniffles or are re-ally seriously ill, the baseline Healing Cells blood count goes up. Our blood Healing Cells count goes up and down all throughout our lives as it works at healing us, 24 hours every day, 7 days per week … from cradle to grave. At any given time the healing cell system in our bone marrow may be very active as demonstrated by a high Healing Cell blood count and at other times less active, but never stopping.

Do you remember the TV commercials for Roach Hotels … "They can get in, but they can't get out"? Well, Healing Cells are like that.

Once trapped in our fat, Healing Cells can't get out
to heal us.

When they are trapped in fat, since fat is not a particularly active tissue metabolically, the Healing Cells go to sleep, metabolically speaking. They have no need to heal, because they cannot re-spond to the hormonal alert for their help by cytokines released by dying older body cells somewhere in the body. So they go to sleep.

Our body cells age, just like our entire human organism does. In fact, our body aging process is a direct reflection of our cells' aging process. Cells age. Cells get old.

Cells age when they reproduce.

Cells age when they are active.

But cells stay young when they sleep (incubate) in fat.

At five years old you may have had a bad bout with the flu or sore throat. At that time your rising blood levels of Healing Cells were filled with a five-year-old's vigor (measurable by reproduction and cytokine production rates which vary exponentially between young and old healing cells). Your vigorous Healing Cells blood count went way up to heal your dying tonsil cells and all the other cell casualties you faced as you were sick in bed at that age. Every time the Healing Cells blood count goes up many more of them have access to fat tissue, so there is a greater chance for more of them to get trapped in fat, and they do.

Lots of those vigorous, youthful five-year-old Healing Cells got trapped (sequestered) in your body fat tissue while you were in your sick bed, home from school. Those young fat-trapped healing cells immediately went to sleep (incubating, stopped reproducing, trans-differentiating, making cytokines or reacting to ambient cytokine hormonal signals.) Those baby-like powerful Healing Cells are still sleeping in your body fat tissue today. We have Healing Cells that went to sleep and stopped aging that got trapped in our fat when we were all one year old, two years old, three years old, etc., all the way up to our current age.

These sleeping Healing Cells, if clinically un-trapped from their fat tissue slumber and released into the blood, are exponentially more active than any bone marrow derived healing cell taken from the same older patient (say 50 years old).

As fanciful as it may sound it is rather medically accurate to say that our natural Healing Cells organ system has been effectively keeping some of our young healing cells young by stashing some away every time there is an abundance of them in our blood throughout life, stashed away and kept physiologically young for us within our bodies' fat adult stem cell sleeping trap.

It is now true that those cells are available to us by simple, safe and easy to perform medical methods. It is as simple as pulling a little fat out of the patient's body (minor liposuction), processing them and injecting the Healing Cells into an arm vein.

"The universe is full of magical things

patiently waiting for our wits to grow sharper."

(Eden Phillpott)

There are specialized cells that also get trapped in fat which are called T-suppressor cells, which are able to suppress the over-active immune system in patients with autoimmune diseases.

There are other specialized Healing Cells called mesenchymal Healing Cells, which decrease inflammation by decreasing in-flammatory cytokines, such as TNF-a (tumor necrosis factor alpha) as well as increasing anti-inflammatory cytokines such as IL-10 (interleukin 10).

Because these particular effects occur rapidly, we have witnessed patients with so much inflammatory rheumatoid arthritis that they were unable to walk, who then improved their mobility within mere hours of their own (autologous) liposuction derived fat-released mesenchymal Healing Cells injections into their arm veins.

We know in medical science that patients with autoimmune diseases like MS and rheumatoid arthritis (RA) and many others have an overabundance of immune system attacking T-killer cells in the blood compared with those without autoimmune diseases, as well as having less T-suppressor cells which function to settle down any "overreaction" from an over reactive immune system as seen in all autoimmune diseases. In all autoimmune diseases there is an immune attack on the patient's own tissues with T-killer cells, the synovial tissue of joints in the case of RA and the brain white matter myelin in the case of MS.

Also there are delayed physiologic effects of Mesenchymal Healing Cells, which decrease abnormal inflammation in autoimmune patients by "down regulating" inflammatory T-killer cell number in the blood and "up regulating" anti-inflammatory T-suppressor cell number in the blood.

We believe all these effects come into play in the 40 or so autoimmune multiple sclerosis patients who have been treated in our Central American clinics, now with a nearly 80 percent favorable clinical response rate for significant neurological status improvements, when we use our newest fat-derived autologous cell transplantation protocols.

One of the distinct advantages to fat-derived autologous Healing Cells treatments is the fact that healing cell treatments of any kind have proven to be **very cell number dose dependent**.

When the China clinic doctors visited our Central American clinics we exchanged medical insights, and cell number dose dependents was one of the medical cell treatment notions that they had demonstrated for the world, in my opinion.

So we and others have now shown that the more healing cells of the right variety administered to any patient produces a better clinical result than less of the same cell types (phenotypes).

Because healing cells are accumulating in our body fat for our whole lives, the numbers of healing cells of all kinds available from even a little fat is staggering. A fairly good dose for a healing cell treatment is anywhere from 10 million to 100 million cells. Even from a small liposuction sample there are hundreds upon hundreds of millions of healing cells available as well as T-suppressor cells. So the treatment cell dosages in autologous fat-derived healing cell treatments can be easily and inexpensively kept favorably high in fat-derived healing cell treatments.

The presence of telomerase in healing cells is largely responsible for their profoundly powerful medical use potential.

> Remember: Telomerase is a substance which diminishes cellular aging by protecting DNA telomere length of replicating cells, a substance that must exist naturally in a cell as science cannot artificially put it in a cell safely.

Cell expansion tissue culture bio-technology is about to boom because of the exponential duplication potential of these healing cells. The door to a profoundly powerful, inexpensive, generic healing medical therapeutic tool of awesome potential is now for the first time in medical history open to us, potentially.

I cannot overemphasize how huge this discovery is to the health of people everywhere and to the price tag of American medicine.

We have found for the first time in human history an inborn Healing Cells system. I predict unequivocally that Healing Cells therapeutics cannot help but revolutionize world medicine within a very short time, but only after the world's doctors begin to focus on it as a primary medical remedy, which is not occurring to any reasonable extent so far.

Augmentation

In medical science it is typical in virtually all forms of therapy to use what is called augmentation.

The body is always trying to heal itself. Medical therapy is aimed at helping the body heal itself by augmenting the healing process by all medical means known and available. That in a nutshell is all of medical therapeutics.

We augment the immune system with vaccines to fight off certain infections.

We augment our natural anti-bacterial process by adding penicillin antibiotics.

We augment healing from a tumor or abscess by removing it surgically.

We administer molecules, drugs to augment the body's blood pressure homeostasis, or our blood cholesterol homeostasis, or our body's sleep mechanism, etc.

Augmentation is how medical therapy works. We learn a high level of scientific understanding of how the human body works, and then augment some defense against the ravages of diseases.

All that I claim in this book is that there is an intricate, complex, interwoven healing cellular system that we have discovered. We must now learn about it quickly, which we are able to do easily if we focus on it. We must learn everything about how this totally natural cell healing system works so we can use the many ways there are going to be without doubt to medically augment the complex physiological activities of the human Healing Cells organ system.

So far we have learned that 1) we can release healing cells from fat, 2) we can expand their numbers because they are more effective in large doses, 3) we can add drugs that assist them, 4) we can learn when the most effective time in the course of each disease is best to administer them, and 5) we can learn which combinations of the different healing cells are most effective with each of the many diseases we learn to treat. We have already started this very safe and easy process, using well accepted medical methodologies in Central America. I'm not saying all overseas clinics are good the way we were, as we were using the highest standards of safe medical practice.

Every patient treated properly the world over adds important information to solve the medical puzzle of the 21st Century.

The greening of modern medicine

Healing Cells treatments are "green medicine," because these Healing Cells are a powerful natural resource which is normally thrown away as bio-waste, a waste of enormous potentially recyclable, expandable by known safe medical methodologies, usable American healing medical energy.

Just as fossil fuel contains biologically stored usable energy, so too do these cells contain stored natural therapeutic healing energy which is likewise biologically endowed.

We throw these cells away instead of using them, these cells that have harnessed usable medical energy to heal, a healing ability stored within a complex set of biological functions which are encoded and activated genetically within our body Healing Cells' DNA.

It took the human race millennia to develop this ancient DNA code that biologically enables certain of our cells to heal. That is an important fact for mankind to focus on with our proven collective brilliance in science.

We would be wise to stop throwing away this valuable biological cell healing energy that could be safely expanded exponentially in our medical laboratories by current medical methods and then used safely in our American clinics to fuel our health and vitality.

We could eliminate less energy-efficient medical therapies that sap our national resources because they are less effective and more expensive. Put quite simply, by using these cells clinically to recycle their healing energy instead of wasting it would be the greening of modern medicine in our world.

Natural food is all the rage

We continue to see natural food stores popping up in ever increasing numbers and popularity in the USA today. The natural garden outside the White House planted by the First Lady and her children has gotten wide publicity and general approval. Why is the First Lady advocating natural garden food for the First Family's dinner table and even for us? Why do some in our

American culture recommend unprocessed, unadulterated natural foods for best health?

Is such a strong preference for unadulterated natural forms of food instead of processed or otherwise man-altered food really a scientifically valid medical and public health notion?

Could it be based on myth or more cynically, a hyped-up natural and organic food industry vying for profits? Are the First Lady and many other Americans being fooled by the American "natural food craze"? If natural food is actually better for our health, why would it be better?

> "All truths are easy to understand once they are
>
> discovered;
>
> the point is to discover them."
>
> (Galileo)

We all learned in high school that DNA (genetic code) is the super-molecule that controls all multicellular physiology on this planet. No one doubts that in science. All life comes from pre-existing life because all DNA comes from pre-existing DNA.

We cannot change our genes, nor can we change our digestive systems or any other component of our intrinsic physiology because they are held within our nature in a relatively fixed state as dictated by our DNA genetic code.

A food or substance usually proves to be healthy, if and only if, we as a species have been exposed to it during the millions of years our ancestors were evolving.

Science has repeatedly demonstrated that any deviation from our natural diet will and does poison the human body. Processed sugar is the quintessential example. The sugar contained in natural food is in the exact form that humans have been exposed to it since our DNA was evolving. The part of our DNA that controls the details of how our human bodies digest and metabolize sugar started to develop roughly about 4,000 million years ago when the first DNA molecule made its entrance on planet Earth.

That DNA has been evolving and adapting over the millennia to be passed down to the approximate 7 billion humans that are living on the planet today.

It is our DNA that determines what will be a poison and what will be healthy for us.

Our DNA, or put more precisely, our human gene pool can and does adapt and change, but it takes eons of time for such adaptations. Man-altered processed sugar has been with us no more than 200 years.

Even though humans have been exposed to processed sugar for these many years now within our modern life, two hundred years is a statistically irrelevant duration of time when compared, as it should be compared, with the full human evolutionary timeline of human DNA. A mere two hundred years is meaningless and effectively irrelevant to the human DNA gene pool under the population dynamics of that same gene pool over the past 200 years.

Permanent human gene pool DNA adaptations do not occur fast enough to accommodate exposures to new substances in 200 years without near-extinction selective survival dynamics.

Two hundred years is only 1/20,000,000 of our human DNA developmental timeline.

Processed sugar was not "normal" or "usual" or "natural" in the human diet before 200 years ago; therefore, processed sugar is **unnatural and novel** to our DNA-controlled complex physiology and metabolism.

A novel substance to our human bodies is a poison, almost by scientific definition. Our innate DNA controlled natural physiology is not prepared to handle foods containing processed sugar precisely because our bodies have evolved without exposure and evolutionary DNA adaptation to it.

It is actually the "novelty" of substances that make them poison to us (our DNA-controlled systems).

Our ability to metabolize any substance is based on our preexisting DNA code. American children of today are being progressively poisoned by man-altered processed sugar, a form of sugar that has been in existence now for at most 200 years.

Our American industrial scientists have taken simple glucose molecules out of their natural state inside natural plant long molecular carbohydrates, a brutally unscientific medical idea. That action is poisoning our children and us by creating an ever-escalating American national epidemic of type II diabetes mellitus and obesity that we suffer from today, with all their profound and widespread attendant health detriments to our American citizens.

The processed sugar human poison
In response to dietary exposure to high processed sugar intake, humans are essentially poisoned because in response to it our bodies' insulin hormone levels are stimulated to rise faster and

higher than when we eat any natural food; a fact that has terrible, unintended health consequences.

The processed sugar-induced high insulin hormone level in the blood in turn over stimulates the part of our body's trillions of cells that "read the insulin hormonal signal" (somatic cell insulin receptors) throughout our body, which in turn respond by ignoring the insulin hormonal bio-chemical signal in an unsuccessful attempt to re-establish blood sugar balance (blood glucose homeostasis) in a condition called **insulin resistance**; something never experienced when we ate our sugar from normal long carbohydrate molecules found in our pre-modern, natural diet (hunter-gatherer diet).

As the increasing insulin signal is ignored more and more by all the body cells (increasing insulin resistance) the pancreas is forced to produce more and more insulin hormone in a feeble attempt to overcome the fact that all the body cells are ignoring the insulin hormone signal, which keeps the blood sugar level high, which in turn stimulates more insulin production in a processed sugar induced vicious-cycle metabolic disease state, something that never happens with a natural human diet free of processed sugar.

Moreover the abnormally high insulin levels are inflammatory systemically (actually increases an important inflammatory clinical marker, CRP, C-reactive protein) which accelerates all inflammatory degenerative diseases, of which there are many including of course, the biggest killer of Americans, atherosclerosis.

"When one tugs at a single thing in nature,

he finds it attached to the rest of the world."

(John Muir)

This gets so bad that the pancreatic cells have to produce so much insulin that the process kills the insulin-producing cells of the pancreas; they just drop dead from years of overwork, work our genes have not prepared them to do so much of, so they start dropping like flies.

The processed novel sugar in our modern abnormal diet "work to death" our insulin-making pancreas cells. This, of course, leads to what we doctors call full-blown, insulin-dependent type 2 diabetes mellitus, a huge current epidemic, a serious and expensive medical problem for millions of Americans—an epidemic caused by a poison—manmade unnatural novel processed sugar. This also caused our obesity epidemic in America.

"Until man duplicates a blade of grass,

nature can laugh at his so-called scientific know-

ledge."

(Thomas Edison)

The irony is that something as apparently benign as sugar can be a poison to any organism, including humans, that are not exposed to it as part of its evolutionary pathway and evolutionary gene encoded adaptive adjustments.

This is the exact same reason we can't safely eat rubber, nylon, plastic or manmade trans-fatty acids in margarine, either, because all these unnatural substances are poisons to our bodies because their man-altered molecular forms are new to us (novel).

New, **novel**, and **different** is bad for our bodies, practically by definition.

That is essentially why our unadulterated natural diet (normal hunter-gatherer diet) will always be healthier for humans. Natural substances are intrinsically better for human beings because our fixed genetic code compels our physiology to react to unnatural (novel) foreign substances adversely, even if it is as benign sounding as sugar.

The notion that **natural is healthier for a human being** is not only true, it is a well-established and profound scientific truth. That natural is healthier for human beings cuts to and drills down to the very core, the heart and soul of a major primary medical and scientific principal. The notion that natural is healthier for a human is a medical truth of great and enduring value to mankind. It is among many other things a message from the graves of Drs. Jenner, Fleming, Einstein and many others.

Medical science is nature.

Medical science is nature explained and understood.

Nature is the source of medical scientific information.

> "An experiment is a question which science poses
> to Nature, and a measurement is the recording of
> Nature's answer."
>
> (Max Planck)

Roger M. Nocera, M.D.

Many Americans have come to believe that nature is somehow unimportant in our high tech modern lives and in health and in high tech human medicine.

These are thoughts which we entertain at our peril. Nature has always proven supreme in science, medicine, and health. All the great medical discoveries that have changed the world dramatically and enduringly were only about one thing ... nature, because only through nature can medical science and all science advance.

"Man, being the servant and interpreter of nature,

can do and understand so much and so much only

as he has observed in fact or in thought of the

course of nature:

beyond this, he neither knows anything nor can

do anything."

(Sir Francis Bacon)

CHAPTER FOUR

OUR "UN-NATURAL" MEDICAL PARADIGM

"Hell is truth seen too late."

(Thomas Hobbes)

American medicine is sick

I am not the first person to declare out loud that our American medical healthcare system is ailing and broken. It seems to be a well accepted fact, although American consensus is polarized on the solutions to fix the problem.

What is clear is that no country can continue to survive or properly serve its citizens, let alone thrive and create needed new jobs, while paying 18 percent of its Gross Domestic Product (GDP) for its healthcare, especially when 18 percent of GDP is taken off the top of nearly all American industry profits. Moreover, that worldwide unprecedented expense level continues to rise unabated as it has for many decades.

Common sense dictates that we cannot compete in a global economy in which the next most expensive country pays only 11 percent of GDP for their healthcare, with all the rest having price tags that shrink rapidly thereafter.

That next most expensive country (France) and all others not only pay a fraction of what we Americans pay for healthcare but, as if to add insult to injury, most of these countries have been shown in a comprehensive scientific analysis conducted by the World Health Organization to enjoy far better and more effective medical care than we Americans do, by a very wide margin, as reflected in virtually every objective, evidence-based, medical healthcare outcome index measurement known to modern medical epidemiology.

In other words, in comparison to the rest of the world, we Americans have been scientifically documented to be paying more and more to get less and less effective healthcare. As a trained medical diagnostician I am compelled to view these facts as merely symptoms of an underlying primary causative problem, hidden from sight, percolating maliciously beneath the surface, operating within the bowels of our American medical healthcare industry, a 2.4 trillion dollar per annum colossus which is admittedly broken.

Our medical system is sick, and although we think we know what is causing our malady, we really don't.

America's diagnosis of our healthcare system's ailment is incorrect, which explains why no one has been able to fix it, either now or for all the decades it has been known to be perniciously incubating.

America's political polarities as well as the shrinking population in between them always ultimately focus on perusing solutions to America's healthcare cost crisis that are some variation in how we pay out money for healthcare.

The global American idea seems to be that if we could just "pay" for healthcare in just the right way our problem would be over.

Conceptually we have all accepted that the answer is hiding in the sum and substance of the details of the way we pay for healthcare in America.

And there are no shortages of divergent variations on the way-to-pay theme. Most Americans seem to be passionately sure that the answer to our healthcare problem is fixing how we pay for it.

It is not.

The real problem is that our doctors have absolutely no say whatsoever about what therapies they have to offer us when we get sick.

What we **must not do** is only treat symptoms of this problem, rather than treating the cause. Treating symptoms rather than causes is an ancient therapeutic folly, a trap that can lead to a medical misadventure and potentially a bottomless pit of increasingly expensive and ineffective temporizing "cures."

American science is sick?

The actual cause of American's healthcare system ailment is the pathologic manner in which America conducts medical scientific research and not how we pay for retail health care.

Our problem can only be accurately analyzed, understood and then rapidly corrected from a national scientific research perspective.

American medical science is literally making us sick. It is medical science that is broken in America, and has been broken for a long time.

The pathologic impact of the nation's defective medical science system is about to intensify, and further metastasize systemically, possibly precipitating a full blown economic collapse, if something is not done quickly.

We need to understand unequivocally and in accurate detail how our medical science research system is broken and then we need a specific plan to fix it based on changing the actual factors that are perpetuating the illness in our system.

"To be gravely regarded"

Healthcare is often considered by economists to be a non-productive industry because the cost to any nation spent to maintain the health of its citizens, while desirable and important, produces no actual product for international commerce and is considered an economic drain because it adds nothing directly to a nation's actual wealth.

The percentage of our GDP spent for healthcare has been increasing for decades and continues to increase at a faster rate than the GDP itself. One does not need a Ph.D. in economics to realize that this continued acceleration in costs relative to our GDP is unsustainable.

We pay more per capita for our healthcare than any other country, by a huge factor.

Because we spend vastly more than any other country for our healthcare many proud Americans believe that this extra expenditure assures us that ours is the best healthcare in the world, ostensibly an enviable circumstance.

I have often heard many intelligent, apparently thoughtful Americans claim that our American medical practices are clearly superior when compared with other countries, perhaps all other countries. Yet, in fact, all the objective epidemiological evidence on the subject clearly indicates that nothing could be further from the truth.

The World Health Organization 2000 comparative analysis of the world's healthcare systems, ranked by epidemiologically analyzed medical performance and the health of their citizens, did not demonstrate U.S. superiority. In fact, we did quite dreadfully.

In the category of our U.S. citizens' overall level of health, corrected for age, an objective outcome-based parameter of any national healthcare system's effectiveness, the **U.S. ranked 72nd**! That's correct—there are 71 countries whose citizens are healthier than ours according to the WHO epidemiological health care study.

It was not much better news in our medical system's disease specific outcome performance ranking, which placed us 37th in the world, behind 36 other countries, many of which Americans commonly believe are less sophisticated and less advanced technically than the U.S.

We spend much more than any other country for healthcare, yet our healthcare performance and citizens' health have been objectively measured and declared inferior to countries spending much less per capita! Clearly, something is not right.

The exchange rate within our current U.S. healthcare system, between dollars spent for health and the actual health achieved is "out of whack." We just aren't getting health value for our dollars.

A strong voice from the past
The culprits for this disconnect between medical cost and medical performance in America is a flaw in American scientific research.

In what has been dubbed his "vast military industrial complex speech," President Dwight D. Eisenhower brilliantly attempted to warn our nation's citizens that we had a flaw in how scientific research was conducted in our country.

The no-nonsense hero of World War II, Supreme Commander of our NATO forces in Europe, four star General and former two term President of the United States was clearly no hysterical alarmist when he emphasized that the flaw in American science was to be "gravely regarded."

President Eisenhower was hauntingly correct in his farewell speech to the nation from The White House where he presented his articulate, sage analysis and his grave public warning about his concerns of how America conducts scientific research, an extraordinary warning spoken by a great leader, yet his admonition has unfortunately been sitting on the mantle, collecting dust, unheeded for fifty years now.

The discovery process in medical science research has been disrupted since Eisenhower issued his fateful warning, and the flaw in science of which he spoke has been negatively impacting our waywardly growing medical industry ever since, as it continues to do today (the president's exact words to come).

The pathway for this national pathology is that bad science leads to less efficacious yet more costly medical treatments and procedures.

Imagine a problem in our medical system that cannot help but continuously increase costs for medical care while producing ever less effective medical practices. Because of the way our medical science system operates new medical inventions cost more and more but are ever more disappointing therapeutically.

That is the medical system we have and why this system is doomed to failure as Eisenhower warned us fifty years ago. President Eisenhower issued a poignant warning about the high costs associated with scientific research that had become so expensive, even in his time, that he believed scientists were losing their intellectual freedom. He warned us that formerly independent American universities had become controlled by big money projects that took away scientific free thought, intellectual curiosity and scientific freedom. He warned us of grave consequences arising from the ongoing domination of the nation's scholars by big money interests.

Of course, there has been over a half century of exacerbation and accumulation of negative effects from the influence of big money on scientific research in our country since President Eisenhower spoke these profound prognostic words on the subject in his farewell address to the American people:

> Research has become central; it also becomes more formalized, complex, and costly. ... Today, the solitary inventor, tinkering in his shop, has been overshadowed by task forces of scientists in laboratories and testing fields. In the same fashion, the free university, historically the fountainhead of free ideas and scientific discovery, has experienced a revolution in the conduct of research. Partly because of the huge costs involved, a... contract becomes virtually a substitute for intellectual curiosity. For every old blackboard there are now hundreds of new electronic computers. **The prospect of domination of the nation's scholars by ... project allocations, and the power of money is ever present – and is gravely to be regarded.** Yet, in holding scientific research and discovery in respect, as we should, we must also be alert to the equal and opposite danger that **public policy could itself become the captive of a scientific-technological elite.**
>
> It is the task of statesmanship to mold, to balance, and to integrate these and other forces, new and old, within the principles of our democratic system – ever aiming toward the supreme goals of our free society.
>
> (President Eisenhower)

Despite this explicit and implicit warning by President Eisenhower our country has allowed big money interests to kidnap all American medical scientific freedom and relegated the U.S.'s medical army of Ph.D. medical scientists, researchers and all medical doctors to mere dominated pawns in our national medical research system. Therefore, by extension, **those Eisenhower "big money interests" dominate our entire American healthcare system by controlling medical science, which dictates what our medical doctors can offer us for therapy when we get sick.**

Our national, grave problem in scientific research was inadvertently predestined to lead us exactly where we find ourselves today: spending too much for high-tech medical therapy but getting precious little improvement in our health.

This pathologic situation is apparently not understood by anyone speaking out in the news or in Congress in either political party, or the executive branch during our country's recent "great" debate on the subject, as I have never heard anyone discuss this factor.

This "Eisenhower flawed science factor" has created our American healthcare cost crisis because the flaw in science of which the President spoke created therapies over time that are impressive appearing on the surface, highly technological, enormously expensive, yet they simply do not work very well (as you will see).

The role of the FDA and the USA patent protection system

The FDA requires that any new medical therapeutic device or substance be proven both safe and effective. The burden of proof, with its attendant cost, lies with the entity proposing the new medical therapy for development.

In modern times the costs required to develop a new therapy and prove that it is both safe and effective runs into the hundreds of millions of dollars, an escalating cost that put scientists and doctors out of control of the process entirely, unless they happen to have a few hundreds of million dollars in their personal treasure chest.

Anyone providing this huge amount of funding would have no incentive to do so without some kind of patent protection, which would be necessary to recuperate this gargantuan amount of investment dollars, as well as a reasonable profit.

If there were no patent protection for such a therapy, as soon as the FDA approved it, everyone would be allowed to use it freely and the investors of the hundreds of millions of dollars would lose their investment. They are not going to let that happen. That's not how our system works.

The U.S. patent system was devised to encourage innovation, which has clearly propelled our country into the forefront of the world's economies for decades. The good intentions and past successes of our U.S. patent protection system are apparent, especially in non-medical fields.

However, a patent system based on **novelty** in medicine encourages unnatural therapeutics, which of necessity eventually ruins any medical system over time.

The laws of man and the laws of human biology have collided in the U.S. patent courts.

A therapy is patentable only if it is **new**.

The verbiage used for this patent criterion of newness is "**novel-ty**."

A therapeutic device or substance must be novel to be patentable, yet if something is found within nature it cannot, generally speaking, be considered novel by U.S. patent law; or worse, it is risky to defend as novel in U.S. patent court.

If one were to invent a novel way to extract something from nature then a novel process of extraction may be patent-defendable and perhaps a de facto patent on the natural substance itself; but only if the extraction process is a limiting factor in the production of the new therapeutic product, and usually it is not.

If however, something natural has therapeutic benefit but there is no novel way to extract it, then it will be relatively impossible to defend a patent protection claim to it in U.S. patent system and courts. One may certainly try to patent protect a natural product, but to do so requires spending tens of millions or often hundreds of millions of dollars, which would be required to defend such a patent protection claim in our U.S. patent court system, and the courts may very well rule against you.

This exorbitant and often prohibitively expensive patent protection legal process leaves all scientists desperate for the huge funding needed to develop any new therapy, a process of monumental importance and huge costs of its own. Certainly, Wall Street knows before they fund any new medical therapy idea, it had better be clear that the therapy involves a novel invention according to U.S. Patent Law, or funding its development would be unwise, to say the least.

Because a natural therapy is relatively un-patentable in the U.S. for all practical purposes, coupled with the astronomical costs of modern, double-blind, placebo-controlled medical research, the U.S. medical research industry has been inadvertently compelled to create ever more unnatural, novel therapeutics.

This artificial, novelty-propelled market force profoundly affects the focus of our country's medical researchers, favoring unnatural therapy development.

The US patent system has uncoupled science from nature

The proper focus of medical research, however, is a medical consideration, not an economic one.

"No one should approach the temple of science

with the soul of a money changer."

(Thomas Browne)

The current American therapeutic paradigm, which has developed within our country during decades of exposure to the novelty requirement of our research system, has become increasingly replete with synthetic, unnatural and highly technical therapeutics, forever novel but increasingly more expensive, technical and ineffective.

Therapeutic bio-chemicals found in nature can be patent-protected in our system only if they can be "de-naturalized" bio-chemically, and of course that is always easy to do with current bio-chemical technology.

Mind you, the natural versions may be exponentially better than the synthetic copies, but that only devalues the bio-chemical in the eyes of those researchers dominated by "big money interests" who are interested first in patent protection, second in safety, and third in effectiveness.

There are many drugs on the market today, which are manmade synthetic renditions of natural substances that have been made unnatural in order to make them patentable.

This is done even if the chemical changes to the natural substance make it more toxic, which they usually do.

Synthetic, unnatural substances do not have to compete with natural ones in our medical system because the latter are not even in the "game." No one will develop medical therapies with them. In our system, less toxic natural substances must be converted with biotechnology into patentable synthetic novel substances that often prove to be more toxic than the natural un-patentable substances which are never clinically tested because of the high costs of such testing. Who would pay for it?

Drugs on the market today are mostly synthetic because they are the most patentable in our system. These synthetic substances are all sold with an obligatory list of adverse side effects—and the side effects are real, and predictable, because as in the example of raw sugar's danger to the human body, all unnatural substances are foreign, and often toxic to the human body.

How many warnings are necessary for an apple, or an orange, unless they have a manmade, patentable synthetic pesticide on them?

The typical drug advertisement on television includes images of the usual gratuitous beautiful people running healthily through lovely natural fields with their happy faces reflecting the sheer joy of using the advertised drug. Toward the end of the advertisement we hear a compendium of horrible sounding potential side effects stated in a tone of voice as though something good were being announced.

These side effects are nothing more than adverse reactions to unnatural substances.

If medical thinking was uninfluenced by non-medical concerns, natural substances would be the focus of medical pharmacology. But that is not the case. In fact, the pharmaceutical lobby has conditioned the population to roll their eyes if they even hear the word natural. "Natural" is code for "ineffective" according to those in control of the billions of investment dollars, and anyone who talks about the benefits of natural products or therapies is portrayed as a gray-haired, pony-tailed, granola muncher.

In our research system, because of the patent protection requirements needed to cover the huge costs of medical research investments, there is often a conflict of interest between the goals of good healthcare and the ability to afford to do the research necessary to bring a therapy to market.

Without "novelty" there is no potential for a new therapy in our system. But as we discussed in previous chapters, nature is the core of all science, but especially in medical science as we humans are products of nature.

Our U.S. patent system "uncoupled" American medical science from a focus on nature and replaced it with a focus on novelty.

Eisenhower warned us that science could easily become uncoupled from the wellbeing of Americans, which is exactly what happened to us, by our own hand, unconsciously and inadvertently. That is why our American healthcare cost crisis problem has been so difficult to diagnose properly. The problem is a deep and grave flaw in our science system.

Our entire American healthcare cost crisis is collectively a set of inevitable symptoms of a flawed system that uncouples medical science from nature.

Potentially wonderful natural therapies wither and die on the vine due to neglect and atrophy because our system requires huge funds to drive the research needed to demonstrate therapeutic efficacy and safety.

Without patent protection a new therapeutic idea in our modern times cannot be investigated; ergo, in the realm of potential new therapeutics, natural has become synonymous with un-patentable, un-researchable and un-doable.

Moreover, the fundamental principles of medical biology clearly portend that as medical therapeutics become ever more unnatural, they also, of necessity, become less effective and more toxic.

My diagnosis is, therefore, that our country's healthcare malady has nothing directly to do with how we pay for healthcare.

Our American healthcare is artificially based on novelty instead of nature, and that is our problem's core. Remove that and health will follow as no other action will or can.

Over the latter half of the 20th Century American healthcare has developed under the unrelenting influence of the following mega-trends:

- astronomically high costs of medical research recoverable only if patent-protected;

- a novelty requirement in the one industry in which it decreases product value;

- a citizenry entirely uneducated about the real medical value of available therapies.

The resultant medical therapeutic paradigm in America today is unnatural, synthetic, mechanical, high-tech, ridiculously expensive, impressive to watch, and largely ineffective.

Alternative medicine

A few decades ago, due to the high-tech, unnatural trend in medical therapeutics, many patients and doctors sought something more natural, less synthetic, less toxic and less painful and invasive, leading to the development of naturopathic, alternative, and holistic medical paradigms in the U.S.

New types of medical schools were developed in formal protest to the denaturalized processes in conventional M.D. medicine (allopathic medicine).

However, the new alternative medical paradigms have remained limited because alternative medical therapeutics are so natural as to be completely un-patentable and any attempt to patent these therapies would be immensely expensive and financially risky.

Therefore, we have not seen any serious development of much alternative medical therapeutics.

Medical therapeutics, the kind that advances mankind, is established by research, very costly research, without which no therapeutic paradigm can evolve in modern times. Without research, therapeutic success is at best anecdotal, a dirty word in conventional allopathic medical realms. The effect of the novelty requirement of our patent system coupled with the exorbitant costs required for research and the legal defense of patent claims has created a dysfunctional medical system, which is synthetic, unnatural, high-tech, exorbitantly expensive, and yes, impressive but often ineffective.

Our system expends far too much monetary and human energy for the amount of healing it provides. That is the essence of our healthcare cost crisis.

After spending enormous amounts of money and human effort for healthcare, we remain sick. This is exactly where we are today. The WHO 2000 study has demonstrated that we Americans are less healthy than other countries' citizens despite our greater expense for higher technology healthcare. With a system like this, no amount of spending or special system of payments will make us well. No amount of congressional action to change medical care reimbursement regulations could possibly fix this problem, nor even approach addressing the problem, be they multiple payers, single payers, private or socialized methodologies.

Only a fundamental paradigm shift in medical therapeutics can avert further dysfunction and further deviation from nature and health.

Only a therapeutic paradigm shift to a more natural realm will save us from the exorbitant costs of our ineffectual, unnatural, high-tech therapeutic American medical system.

Roger M. Nocera, M.D.

It has many whistles and bells, but does very little

At this point it may be illuminating to present a few examples of commonly employed high-tech medical paradigm therapies, their cost and health results. I have picked examples that are emblematic of the high- tech medicine problem as I see it.

The first is the surgery that is commonly performed in the U.S. on patients having a high risk for strokes . . . "an artery in your neck clean-out surgery" (a carotid endarterectomy).

A stroke is a rapid loss of brain function due to a disturbance in blood supply. Most strokes occur because of a buildup of fatty cement (atherosclerotic plaque) on the walls of the arteries in the neck which feed the brain blood (carotid arteries). The arterial wall fatty cement predisposes these blood vessels to develop blood clots.

The vast majority of strokes in America occur from a process whereby one of these blood clots breaks free (thromboembolism) and flows with the blood through the arteries of the brain until it creates an obstruction to blood flow causing loss of blood delivery and death (ischemic) to a part of the brain . . . a typical stroke.

Our high-tech medical paradigm has little to offer anyone therapeutically once a stroke has occurred. Therefore, prevention of strokes is the purpose for an artery in your neck clean-out surgery (carotid endarterectomy).

This is why physicians listen to their patients' necks with stethoscopes.

They are listening for a characteristic rattling of high velocity blood (a bruit) as it passes through the arteries that are narrowed by the fatty cement on the walls of the arteries feeding the brain.

When a doctor hears this rattling in a patient's neck with her stethoscope the standard of care requires her to evaluate further with an ultrasound (Doppler and real time), and possibly a picture of the arteries with an MRI (a magnetic resonance arteriogram and eventually a catheter carotid arteriogram).

Once enough artery fatty cement is identified by these tests and is deemed to be dangerous for future strokes (a hemodynamically significant carotid stenosis), the next step is an artery in your neck clean-out (a carotid endarterectomy), a surgery in which the neck is cut open, the carotid artery feeding your brain is cut open and the fatty cement (atherosclerotic plaque) is removed.

Patients hate it, of course, but it's worth the pain and risk—right?

So how well does an artery in your neck clean-out surgery (a carotid endarterectomy) actually work and how much health benefit has this surgery given the American people during the past three decades or so?

The answer is: up to 12 percent.[109, 110, 111, 112, 113, 114]

Yes - "up to" 12 percent of all the patients who have received this dangerous, scary surgery over the past few decades have benefited more than they would have with conservative non-surgical treatment using inexpensive mild anticoagulation such as aspirin. The up to 12 percent who benefit statistically, benefit by living a few more years without a stroke than those that do not have the surgery but instead take only aspirin.

These statistics indicate that at least 88 percent of an artery in the neck clean- out surgery patients (carotid endarterectomy patients) who undergo this costly, risky and painful high-tech medical therapeutic intervention do not benefit at all.

Worse yet, some studies have shown that in certain patients the surgery will statistically shorten their lives, and some die during surgery, an elective preventative procedure (prophylactic).

Moreover, there are studies indicating that while these surgeries have been shown to have up to a 12 percent benefit when they are performed by specialists in large research medical centers, that same 12 percent benefit is more difficult to demonstrate in smaller, less sophisticated community hospitals around the country where doctors don't get to perform the surgery often enough to be as competent as those who do many more of these procedures on a regular basis in major teaching hospitals - hardly an unexpected influence on the therapeutic outcome of such an operator-dependent procedure like vascular surgery.

These statistics indicate that over the last three decades in our country at least 88 percent of endarterectomy surgery patients have paid for all the expensive tests and have endured the invasive surgery with all its attendant pain and problems (morbidity and iatrogenic mortality) without any benefit whatsoever.

This is not a very effective therapy, yet the costs to the American healthcare system are exorbitant in order that it marginally benefit only up to 12 percent of those who receive it.

The evaluation and tests (work up) of the artery in the neck clean-out surgery and the surgery itself (carotid endarterectomy) cost our system about 15,000 dollars per patient, or about 1.5 million dollars for every 100 patients receiving this surgical procedure.

Since only up to 12 patients on average will receive any benefit per 100 surgeries performed, the real cost for this treatment to the American healthcare system, which we all pay for in one way or another, is a whopping 125,000 dollars per successful surgery.

This is not a lot of "bang for the buck" because the therapy is so unnatural as to be medically crude.

Heart Bypass Surgery (a coronary artery bypass graft, CABG)

Another illustrious example of high-tech medicine's ineffectiveness is heart bypass surgery (coronary artery bypass graft, CABG).

Over the last three decades or so in our American medical healthcare system, when a patient has chest pain the "standard of care" requires that a set of tests (a work up) be performed, including a physical examination, perhaps a bicycle stress test with pictures (nuclear medicine image assisted stress cardiolyte scan, replaced thallium scans) and ultimately an arteriogram evaluation (catheter coronary arteriogram).

When sufficient narrowing of the arteries feeding the heart from fatty cement (atherosclerotic plaque) is discovered with these tests an invasive surgery may be performed, which is called a heart bypass (coronary artery bypass graft—CABG).

In this surgery the chest is cut open with an electric saw, the ribs are separated with a clamp, the heart is exposed and grafts of various kinds are sewn into the clogged arteries to bypass the fatty cement-narrowed arteries.

Auspiciously, there are American cardiac institutes dedicated to this serious and certainly impressive surgical procedure. But how much health benefit has this surgery (CABG) given the American people during the past three decades or so? The answer differs according to the studies used to determine it, which have been published in peer review journals from time to time throughout the last few decades

Published statistics indicate that roughly 0 to 13 percent of patients will benefit from this surgery with additional years of life over the statistical outcome that would have occurred if no surgery was performed.[115, 116, 117, 118, 119, 120]

At best, 13 percent of the patients that received this surgery in America over the last few decades lived longer on average than patients with the same amount of disease that did not get the surgery and were instead treated with inexpensive anticoagulants like aspirin.

At least 87 percent of the patients that had their chests literally sawed open for this invasive procedure demonstrated no benefit in extending their lives.

This surgery has been partly supplanted by less invasive treatments that were developed in my first specialty of diagnostic radiology in the division of special procedures; namely, catheter delivered balloon angioplasty and later, stent placements, which have shown improved results in only certain types of cases.

Yet this high-tech procedure, heart bypass surgery (CABG), is being performed in America although these procedures often have marginal long term results.

In fact, the results of this surgery are still being evaluated for different patient groups. Moreover, as in the case of an artery in the neck clean-out (carotid endarterectomy), heart bypass surgery (CABG) also proved to be worse than non-surgical treatment in certain types of cases.

Both procedures have been shown to cause earlier death statistically in some patients with certain types of atherosclerosis disease configurations as compared with inexpensive non-surgical treatment.

The most optimistic view is that as many as 13 percent of patients having a heart bypass surgery will live longer than if they do not have this surgery and are treated only with aspirin. Each surgery costs on average 75,000 dollars; therefore, for every 100 patients the cost to the American healthcare system is 7.5 million dollars.

This comes out to be at least 576,000 dollars per successful heart bypass surgery over the past few decades.

Moreover, even the 13 percent of successful patients did not become fully well, but lived somewhat longer in their old age while requiring years of additional medical care, costing the system even more.

There are many other examples of how our modern high-tech medical paradigm has been exorbitantly expensive, yet ineffectual.

Moreover, this statistical analysis of the true benefit of these and many other therapies is not understood by those who receive them as patients because these statistics are not well publicized and are actually hard to find anywhere in our American culture. I have personally asked many patients who have received these high-tech surgical therapies if their doctors informed them of these well-established success and failure statistics. Not one of them has ever said yes. I have never met a patient that was informed of the low percentage of patients that benefit from these risky and painful procedures.

I've also asked a number of doctors who were likewise completely unaware of the dismal statistics on these therapies (CABG and carotid endarterectomy).

These two examples hopefully convey the point that while our current medical practices appear technically impressive, they often fail to deliver as much improved health as splash and glitter, and they are at the very heart of the healthcare cost crisis plaguing our country.

"Of several remedies, the physician should

choose the least sensational."

(Hippocrates)

PART TWO

PREFACE TO PART TWO

"… you will know the truth,

and the truth will make you free."

(John 8:31-32)

I wrote this book for one simple reason. I believed that writing it would help more patients in more medically critical ways than I could accomplish in my customary busy diagnostic medical practice, which I have faithfully engaged in American hospitals and clinics for over thirty years in medicine.

The good medical news is this: a bright new era in health is right at the world's medical science doorway, knocking, sometimes quite loudly. The bad medical news is that this knocking is largely unheard, and therefore unanswered.

Unimaginably wonderful health and economic benefits for us all, including our families, are very close at hand . . . much closer than the public has been led to believe. But we will not harvest those tremendous benefits unless and until we collectively hear, listen to and heed that knocking and open that door together.

Decades from now medical historians will be evaluating the details of events that led to what is about to happen to us next in medicine. They might choose to call the results of these events, many yet to happen, the Great Worldwide Medical Paradigm Shift of the Early Twenty-first Century. For all our sakes, let's hope the coming events compel those medical historians to use that word ... "early."

Here now is the potentially troublesome medical news of which I feel duty bound by my Hippocratic Oath to communicate publically. This section of the book is a public medical alarm of serious gravity, a medical alert in the public square about a preeminent national and worldwide medical problem.

The cause of this grave medical problem remains hidden from the world's public scrutiny, as does the solution which is likewise hidden from public understanding including that of most practicing doctors of medicine and certainly including our government and our politicians.

My premise is that once the cause of this longstanding systemic problem is recognized and understood by the public, both the cause and solution are revealed simultaneously and available to public scrutiny, and therefore, to the influence of medical common sense.

This book is then, by necessity, a "made for the public" medical science lesson, one which is desperately needed. We need a public medical science lesson in common vernacular that everyone can understand, because our American public's medical problem requires a remedy of medical truth, a remedy born of medical understanding, a remedy of accurate medical information based on time tested, well accepted conventional medical principals. It is a remedy that the public will be unfortunately forced to self-prescribe.

It is the nature our medical problem and the hidden solution that requires public scrutiny because our national medical institutions, all of them, have clearly proven to be incapable and highly resistant to do their jobs to resolve for us this worsening medical dilemma.

The bad news is that the non-medical public will have to effectively demand certain needed changes in American medicine because otherwise those needed changes will not happen. Moreover, this medical dilemma has widespread consequences now ripe to crescendo to calamitous proportions, an event that will negatively and profoundly impact all American citizens' health and wealth.

> "The truth will set you free, but first it will make
>
> you miserable."
>
> (President James A. Garfield)

A backward and destructive government regulation
The 2000-DOCS discovery of Healing Cells is being systematically ignored by our American medical industry, a backward-thinking process spawned and enforced by our FDA's ban against American doctors to use this new science in America.

The FDA has banned our American doctors from clinically using these safe, natural Healing Cells to help their ill patients.

The FDA's ban against our doctors remains unquestioned even though they have long since approved the exact same procedure for treating American patients specifically for bone marrow replacement, a therapy that has been carried out safely and legally for decades in America.

The FDA has even forbidden American doctors from using a patient's own natural Healing Cells to help them when they get sick, even though other FDA-allowed therapies use the exact same long standing medical principles that are medically prudent and safe (autologous tissue transplantations).

In other words, for whatever reason you can imagine, our U.S. FDA went out of their way to handle the use of adult stem cells, including fat-derived from the same patient (his own autologous Healing Cells) differently than they had logically in the past. Our FDA is using the regulation methods of drugs to govern adult stem cells use, even our own natural Healing Cells.

What the FDA fails to understand is that the rules of the old molecular therapeutic paradigm (drugs) are insufficient to regulate the higher biological complexity of the new cellular therapeutic paradigm.

What we do in Central America has been made illegal here in America by our FDA. Not because it is dangerous, controversial or unethical. It is hardly different than removing a bit of fat from one area of the body to "plump up" another, or than receiving a blood transfusion from a blood donor. This is nothing less than an assault to every doctor's right to treat his patients according to the medical principals we learned in medical school and teaching hospital residency. Today, doctors know virtually nothing of the discoveries in this book because they have been uncoupled from their medical wisdom and their right to free medical thought and proper medical practices, just as Eisenhower warned. We doctors have been dominated by a scientific technological elite supported by the un-American practices by our own FDA to everyone's great detriment, just as President Eisenhower predicted with uncanny specificity and dread.

Our doctors' medical thoughts are being controlled by uninformed federal government bureaucrats of the FDA.

Many other world cultures depend on the exorbitant expenditures needed for FDA approval in the USA. So many other countries save that money by simply legalizing new treatments only if the big spenders in the USA get FDA approval here. **So when our FDA is wrong it makes many other countries wrong also!**

America's FDA controls a lot of wrong minded "groupthink" about stem cells in our world.

What our FDA must be helped to realize is that American physicians collectively represent a valuable national treasure which it is causing to be underutilized at present.

Our Ph.D. level medical scholars, our American medical doctors, are actually forbidden to use their educations and clinical judgment to help their patients with this new, safe medical science because of the FDA's ill-advised ban on doctors' ability to use this new perfectly safe science.

This untapped and frustrated energy within our American doctors' professional medical minds is a terrible thing to waste. Releasing this pent up medical scholarship and clinical judgment in America would be wise, immediately effective and "green," the correct color of our grandchildren's future.

It is especially frustrating to know that we doctors could begin to use our skills to construct for Americans a more efficient, compassionate and affordable American professional therapeutic medical paradigm.

If our practicing physicians were allowed by the FDA to implement and exploit this new medical science of Healing Cells within our American clinics and hospitals as we have overseas, in a simple, medically-safe and open clinical effort, we could and would expeditiously, safely and inexpensively trigger this much-needed shift in the American medical healthcare system. This shift will improve our healthcare and decrease medical costs precipitously and soon.

This is not pie in the sky.

This change in medical practices could begin immediately and occur completely within a few years if allowed and supported. This generation of citizens including us baby boomers would benefit well within our lifetimes if we will just get moving now.

But the FDA is standing in our way because it arrogantly forbids your doctor from helping you with these safe cells, **even the ones taken from your own body!**

Our FDA forbids these treatments while at the same time they have forced our American doctors to use more invasive, less effective, often toxic and vastly more expensive medical treatments. The FDA says it's okay for your doctor to help you prevent strokes with a surgery that cuts open your neck and has an upside medically of only 11 percent, but your doctor is forbidden to help you use your own fat-trapped Healing Cells to help you if you do suffer a stroke, even though it is a totally safe procedure, safer than the treatment the FDA does approve for the disease.

Is that not medical malpractice?

The FDA approves drugs for MS that cost close to 40 thousand dollars a year per patient, which at best decreases MS attacks by only 30 percent; yet your FDA makes it illegal for your doctor to help you with this terrible disease with your own natural fat-trapped healing cells. It's illegal to use your own cells! It's illegal only because they say it is illegal, not because it's medically unsafe or ineffective, or even immoral or controversial.

I publically call into question the competence of our FDA and raise the issue of their medical malpractice in this matter. I question their medical abilities to do their assigned job of helping our citizens because I question their clinical judgment and their level of knowledge of "stem cell" medicine.

> "Unless we put medical freedom into the Constitution, the time will come when medicine will organize into an undercover dictatorship to restrict the art of healing to one class of men and deny equal privileges to others; the Constitution of the Republic should make a special privilege for medical freedoms as well as religious freedom."
>
> (Benjamin Rush, M.D., a signer of the Declaration of Independence and personal physician to George Washington)

"Yet, in holding scientific research and discovery
in respect, as we should, we must also be alert to
the equal and opposite danger that public policy
could itself become the captive of a scientific-
technological elite. It is the task of statesmanship
to mold, to balance, and to integrate these and
other forces, new and old, within the principles of
our democratic system – ever aiming toward the
supreme goals of our free society."

(President Eisenhower)

If the FDA would drop their medically illogical ban on our doctors to help us with our own fat-trapped healing cells not only could we serve our patients more effectively, but we could also stop draining our national resources with therapies that are not effective, are more expensive, more toxic and painful.

Our FDA needs to put an end to their medical science incompetence on stem cells so they can stop committing medical malpractice on the American people and our children.

Collectively American doctors have finite work time and energy, so if they are kept busy doing complicated but less effective time-consuming FDA approved medical treatments, we all lose.

Let's think about this for a moment.

Let's say you've discovered that under the right conditions natural unpatentable Vitamin C can cure 90 percent of patients having a terrible disease that has no current effective cures available.

Now, let's pretend that at the same time research has found a synthetic patentable new drug that will cure only 10 percent of patients with this disease, although unlike Vitamin C, it's a little toxic and has side effects because it is an unnatural synthetic substance (like processed sugar).

The way our system is set up, the Vitamin C cure will NOT survive, while the 10 percent success rate toxic synthetic cure will quickly get funding and will soon become legal.

Not only will it become legal, but it will be declared the "standard of care," a legal requirement for a certain treatment.

And by the way, government and private insurance companies generally will only pay for treatments within this "standard of care" category, and doctors will be wide open to malpractice suits for using the better natural Vitamin C therapy because they failed to employ the "standard of care."

While this insanity rages on, the Vitamin C treatment will never become established as the treatment of choice, or even see the light of day, because without a patent, the funding for the research cannot and will not materialize. The Vitamin C nontoxic 90 percent effective cure rate treatment cannot, will not, and does not happen in our American medical science system.

Additionally, the owners of the synthetic 10 percent cure will publically blast the Vitamin C cure as unscientific because there were no investors to fund the research (requiring a few hundred million dollars) to demonstrate the scientific proof of the effectiveness of the unpatentable natural substance cure rate.

That's how our American medical research system currently works - a grave problem according to President Eisenhower - and I can only agree.

This is exactly what is happening to Healing Cells.

Therefore, we must find another way to evaluate natural, unpatentable cures; otherwise we are doomed to have 10 percent toxic therapies, which are actually rampant in modern medicine today, all this while our scientific medical scholars are being forced to ignore potentially more effective natural therapies. This is the essence of what people do not understand about our system of medical research.

That is why it is important to understand the level of success of current FDA-approved standard of care treatments, which have some healing benefits which everyone, including most doctors, completely overestimate, as we have seen with carotid endarterectomies and GABG.

The FDA ban on doctors using this safe science is very un-green, unevolved, and has led to a harmful waste of great but finite American resources that we all need.

This overregulation of our doctors by the FDA's medically uninformed government regulatory ban is stopping the progress of medical care in America.

"There is nothing more frightening than active

ignorance."

(Goethe)

We must all help to succeed

Unfortunately, nonmedical people in America will need to get involved in the national discussion that we still need to have about stem cells in this country. But this time we need to get our facts about stem cells straight. How else would the harmful FDA over-regulatory ban on our doctors be eliminated if we don't together insist upon it?

The FDA needs to learn that like all Americans, they have a right to their own medical opinions, but not their own medical facts.

Medical facts are established by hard science, but advances in science don't help us if they are ignored, or worse, forbidden by an incompetent government autocratic bureaucracy wanting to control scientific medical thought in our medical doctors.

> "Humankind is not engaged in a battle between
>
> good and evil;
>
> Rather, we are engaged in a battle between truth
>
> and lies."
>
> (Miguel Ruiz, M.D., a famous brain surgeon)

There are only a few small organizations in the world doing the important advanced medical work in Healing Cells. We and a few other medical professionals have engaged the initial clinical struggle, inconveniently overseas, to demonstrate "the proof of concept" of the healing capacity of the 2000-DOCS' discovery of Healing Cells.

My medical message put simply is that this type of clinical work, which is only being done by a few meager clinics scat-

tered around the world, must become the widespread clinical work of the many.

If this type of clinical work with healing cells now being done by the few indeed actually does become the work of the many, then a paradigm shift in medical science and medical practices will be triggered automatically, leading irresistibly to the massive health and economic benefits our world needs today, especially in the U.S. Moreover, this shift would solve the American health care cost crisis very quickly.

But this needed shift will not happen and cannot happen until and unless certain changes in medicine happen first; changes the public will be forced to effectively demand if we are to enjoy our medical science's earned but denied benefits.

Now it is crucial that the FDA get out of the way and let the many join in our professional medical work in a coordinated approach for our citizens' collective benefit and the future well-being of humanity.

This will not happen by itself. We must make it happen together.

"All that is necessary for the triumph of evil

is that good men do nothing."

(Edmund Burke)

The answer

We now know that there are certain adult stem cells, Healing Cells, which are the human body's natural method of healing itself. This is not speculation, it is now hard scientific medical fact, as certain as the earth is round or the planets orbit around the sun. (I might point out that the powers that be delayed scientists from researching and publishing on those subjects as well—the true nature of our solar system—for many years).

Due to bad scientific practices practically the entire field of natural healing adult stem cell research has been foreclosed in the U.S. by our own FDA, throwing out the baby with the bathwater.

What we must do is lift the FDA general ban on natural Healing Cells treatments and allow certain treatments to occur now that we have a working methodology for Healing Cells.

Healing Cells therapeutics is simple and safe, analogous to those who prepare for an upcoming surgical operation by donating their own blood, having it stored for their own use and receiving that stored blood when it's needed.

Or, one could use the analogy of those who have some fat removed from one part of the body and injected into another. The technology is that simple and we and others have found no harmful side effects.

By preventing doctors from treating patients with this totally safe and effective therapy, the FDA is in effect saying the earth is flat and the sun orbits around it. The FDA is holding up American medical science from proceeding because medical science is trying to evolve in a world that does not recognize that the game has changed due to a new medical scientific discovery.

Our medical science is evolving to a higher level of sophistication; cells. Now that we have discovered this next step in medical science it would be foolhardy to ignore it.

Medicine's future will no longer be a molecular-based drug science; it will be a cell science, which is a more evolved biological level of complexity that we now need to investigate robustly, unhampered by uninformed government functionaries.

Imagine how we would ridicule the governments and societies of 200 years ago if they had banned vaccines (although they did at first, of course), or of 100 years ago if they had likewise banned antibiotic treatment (which didn't take off until it became accepted, which took far too long).

We can no longer afford to ignore natural Healing Cells' use in medical therapy. Many millions of lives will be improved and saved almost immediately if we will act to increase our understanding of the most helpful treatment regimens and utilize the many opportunities to augment and enhance the natural processes of the Healing Cells, as we learn more about it by safely directing their natural healing processes in the clinic and openly share the resultant valuable medical information. **If only our FDA would allow us to.**

> "The scientist is not a person who gives the right answers,
>
> he's one who asks the right questions."
>
> (Claude Lévi-Strauss)

In the first decade of the Twenty-First Century it was first demonstrated scientifically that there are normal, natural cells that we all have inside our bodies that literally are healing our bodies, 24 hours a day, 7 days per week, from cradle to grave, by damaged-cell replacement and natural drug production delivered to our body's tissues and blood from our own natural healing cells that help us when we get sick.

Whenever we get sick or injured, Healing Cells are automatically manufactured in our bone marrow and put naturally into our blood circulation. Then these Healing Cells are directed (hormonally) to collect at the exact site of the cell injury to heal and replace our body's injured cells and release natural drugs to help us get well again.

Clearly, we are only as healthy, no more nor less, than the collective health of our body's cells. Unlike drugs (molecular-based pharmaceuticals), which mono-function in the limited capacity of individual substances within our bodies, Healing Cells actually repair body tissue damage by literally replacing dying, injured and malfunctioning body cells with healthy, robust new ones. Healing Cells also release (secrete) their own host of individual substances (hormonally active cytokines), each as powerful as any single drug but better because they are natural substances, released selectively at just the right time in just the right doses by Healing Cells.

It is as though these special "doctor-cells" had their own well stocked natural medicine cabinets ready for any medical situation. These natural drugs (cytokines) coming from healing cells have been proven scientifically to augment healing when we get sick (trophic effects).

We must break through the resistance of our own current day FDA and our own urban, ivory tower medical experts who, on the whole, have not yet embraced, and indeed have shown great animosity and resistance to accept as true, the undeniably true new scientific medical facts about Healing Cells presented and documented in this book.

Roger M. Nocera, M.D.

CHAPTER FIVE

FOCUS

"What is unsought will go undetected."

(Sophocles)

FOCUS IN MEDICAL RESEARCH

The particular focus of scientific research matters more than most Americans realize because they do not understand how scientific research actually works. Americans also think the choice of focus in scientific research is far more limited than it actually is.

Focus in scientific research is preeminent because there are literally infinite possible directions in which scientific research can focus, each with their distinct trajectories and attendant results.

You cannot focus on everything.

Great medical discoveries don't just happen automatically with the passage of time and the application of generic effort. Great discoveries create improvements in the human condition because of only one thing: They change scientific FOCUS. Focus is not just something in science, it is everything.

Focus is what effectuates great discoveries like human immunity and antibiotics; now it is needed for Healing Cells.

How to find a pearl in the sand (or what looks impressive can be scientific junk)

Imagine you have to find a pearl in the sand which was placed one inch below the surface on a beach the size of a football field.

The most domineering scientist has convinced your team that the best way to find the pearl is to begin counting each grain of sand and also cataloging them according to their fractal geometric class, of which there are 30, which are based on a complex microscopic analysis of each sand grain's shape.

This is the focus of the science to find the pearl.

It is a bad focus, which dooms the scientific process to failure. The focus to sift one and a half inches of the sand with a screen with holes just a bit smaller than the size of the pearl would be a different focus of research. I don't know what you know about fractal geometry but it involves very advanced mathematics. So, the first focus of finding the pearl will appear on one level as very erudite, advanced and impressive, yet, the focus of all this hard work is so flawed that the mathematics, no matter how impressive, become irrelevant.

Yet people are impressed with high mathematics, so if they are impressed enough they may not see the flaw in the focus of the endeavor.

This is exactly how our American medical research system is flawed.

It's not that the ivory tower scientists are not clearly brilliant, but if they are forced to focus (or for whatever reason choose to focus) their research on an ill-fated focus of their subject, no amount of brilliance will lead them to success. Once the focus is set upon the fractal geometry of each sand grain in the search for the beach pearl, the outcome is doomed (you will not find the pearl, not in a cost effective or timely manner), despite how brilliant and complex the fractal geometry mathematics is.

It doesn't matter once the focus is off.

The substantial development of a world changing discovery (already made) may be five years away if a particular focus in research is chosen. Yet, if it takes 100 years for that focus to be taken by the nation's scientists then the discovery will be 105 years away. Focus in medical scientific research matters, because if you focus only to the LEFT forever you will never find something hiding to your RIGHT.

Sharing information

Secrecy runs rampant in medical scientific research today because of the fear that ideas and discoveries will be stolen by competitors (who wish to monopolize the discovery through patent protection), which slows research to a fraction of ideal speed.

By failing to share freely in scientific discourse with investigators of different scientific backgrounds, any research system is paralyzed, as is ours. If everyone must reinvent each wheel in the discovery process because investigators have disincentives to share information, then the process grinds to a crawl, extending the years before Healing Cells treatments will cure diseases and save lives.

Results do not automatically occur in science because a lot of money is spent for it. There is, however, a synergistic, exponential increase in the rate of progress when a lot of researchers openly share their findings, ideas and results.

They share FOCUS.

The momentous discovery of the Healing Cells first published in 2000-DOCS is dying of neglect and resultant atrophy because of a complete lack of coordinated scientific focus. Unless and until doctors and medical scholars consciously focus on leveraging this discovery, our country's high-tech medical paradigm will not shift and our exorbitant and still rising healthcare costs will not abate.

Moreover, all that would be required to get the ball rolling expeditiously would be to convince the FDA to drop its ban on doctors using a patient's own Healing Cells for therapeutics (simple autologous transplantations). Just allow safe therapy with the patients' own healing cells as long as a record of the results is sent to a central database to share the information.

Without any change of infrastructure our nation's doctors could safely advance this medical science exponentially, logarithmically fast, which would be the least expensive pathway to develop Healing Cells therapeutics in our country.

How can doctors focus on something made illegal by the FDA medical thought police?

The FDA ban on doctors' rights to prescribe a patient's own fat-trapped Healing Cells to help them when they get sick is a de facto control of your doctors' medical thoughts.

"Don't focus here," they command. "You are not allowed to focus on Healing Cells science, U.S. doctors."

Is it any wonder that our nation's doctors do not know the information in this book? Why would a doctor focus on something he is not allowed to do? Doctors are too busy and practical for that.

The appropriate role of government in medicine
The President of the United States stated that our national angst over healthcare reform relates to a struggle over an important recurring American issue which poses the questions:

·   What is the appropriate role of government in American society?

·   How big should government be?

·   How much government regulation is best?

We have focused our government regulation question on how much as opposed to which type, how, when, where and why.

I believe President John F. Kennedy said it best in his first televised debate with Richard Nixon:

> "I don't believe in big government, but I
> believe in effective governmental action,
> and I think that's the only way that the
> United States is going to maintain its
> freedom; it's the only way that we're
> going to move ahead. I think we can do
> a better job. I think we're going to have
> to do a better job if we are going to meet
> the responsibilities which time and
> events have placed upon us."

I agree that the healthcare argument should not be over the size of government, but whether government is serving the needs of the people, or conversely, the interests of special powerful interest groups bent on obtaining enormous profits, even if that action significantly reduces human wellbeing and delays human progress.

Indeed, "the responsibilities which time and events have placed upon us" all cry out that we make decisions that will improve the health of Americans and people throughout the world while freeing trillions of dollars that could be better spent elsewhere.

Preventing people's access to their own Healing Cells, which have been proven safe and effective around the rest of the world, may help preserve the profits of conventional medical providers, but it makes these life- and health-saving procedures unavailable to all the rest of us Americans. This is a paradigm shift in a critical clinical arena which is currently being largely ignored for a patient's own Healing Cells therapeutics (autologous Healing Cells transplantations) and completely ignored for afterbirth Healing Cells therapeutics (afterbirth-derived allogeneic Healing Cells).

Essentially, using a patient's own Healing Cells is being viewed by the FDA as though this process represented a new drug requiring all the exorbitantly expensive standard research and FDA approval protocols.

I suspect that the FDA is well intentioned, if not muscle-bound by its historical mandate, but this policy has a hideous, unintended consequence. With great reluctance I must call it medical malpractice because it is hurting peoples' chances for better health and longer life.

The FDA's ill-informed ban stalls indefinitely our much needed medical paradigm shift from exorbitantly expensive high-tech medicine to a far less expensive, less painful, less invasive, more natural and more effective Healing Cells therapeutic paradigm.

> "The truth is found when men are free to pursue
>
> it."
>
> (Franklin D. Roosevelt)

Because using a patient's own Healing Cells is unpatentable, little or no private funding for research will be forthcoming.

Yet lifting the FDA ban on doctors to judiciously utilize a patient's own Healing Cells for their treatment would allow our nation's doctors to discover the potential of these cells without the exorbitant costs of traditional formal FDA required proof-of-efficacy, double blind, placebo-controlled research so important for synthetic drugs but painfully inappropriate when applied to natural healing cell medical science.

Because these cells are completely and utterly harmless (and inoffensive to any political or religious philosophy) there is no legitimate need for this FDA ban, which is delaying our medical evolution toward a less expensive, more natural and more efficacious therapeutic paradigm.

Healing Cells therapeutics will create a paradigm shift of the first order. The only question is when the shift will come, and will it come in time to save our economy from the burden of our country's unprecedented healthcare costs and provide health improvements in time for baby boomers?

WHO'S IN CHARGE?

The enormous costs required to conduct medical research has impacted modern conventional medicine over the past 50 years such that no medical doctor or group of doctors has ever been fully in charge, unconcerned with their employer's profit goals when deciding which types of medical therapies should be focused upon and investigated with research.

Only those who control hundreds of millions of dollars ultimately determine the true focus of medical research in this country.

Doctors of medicine, the only citizens actually qualified to determine the correct direction and focus of medical therapeutic research, are not now nor have they ever been in recent times even remotely in charge of determining that direction and focus in the U.S.

Enter the 2000-DOCS's new scientific discovery, which is clearly as important to the future of mankind as the discoveries of the human immune system (vaccines) and antibiotics.

Tragically, leveraging the discovery of Healing Cells by our nation's scholars is inconsistent with our current medical economic system, since Healing Cells are too completely natural and therefore very difficult, expensive and risky to patent protect. Difficult to patent protect means to traditional American medical technology investors that it is an arena impossible to monopolize and sell at exorbitant prices. This means it is impossible to access the medical research investment dollars needed to develop Healing Cells therapies in the traditional way in our American system. This is actually happening now, and retarding our medical evolution to the next big thing in medical science.

None of the usual medical investors will touch it.

Therefore, Healing Cells remain relatively unexplored by either the mainstream or the elite of our modern medical scientific community who are completely dominated, as Eisenhower predicted, by those who clutch the American scientific research purse strings.

All of the research I'm referring to has nothing to do with proving that Healing Cells treatments are effective or that they pose no harm—this is already known—but that it is necessary for the final treatment information for doctors to know when to administer treatment, how many of each possible combinations and permutations of combinations of cells, and in what order and with which of many possible augmentation techniques for each different disease process.

The good news is that since Healing Cells are so unpatentable there is a monumental opportunity for the government to drastically decrease the cost of our medical care by simply allowing American doctors to be doctors and legally prescribe something they know is utterly harmless, totally innocuous, and quite likely helpful therapeutically for their patients, unlike most of the patented therapies now available to them.

Every disease, not just a few

Exploiting Healing Cells will impact the therapy of every disease, not just the few often mentioned during the usual discussion of "stem cells" in general.

We are going to focus on the original, natural, intrinsic cellular healing system of human life, a genetically endowed, complex organ system operational from cradle to grave.

Because the human body is composed of individual units of life—cells—the ability to replace diseased cell units with new cells and create natural healing drugs that heal us (cytokines) is a therapeutic milestone of unfathomable medical significance. The potential impact on humanity of the Healing Cells discovery is not trumped by the discovery of the immune system or antibiotics, I assure you. To say that we have identified a natural cellular healing system that we can study and exploit to our collective therapeutic benefit is so profound that I cannot begin to express what this discovery potentially means to the health of the human race.

CHAPTER SIX

THE HEALING CELLS "MANHATTAN PROJECT"

"The mark of a good action is that it appears inevitable in retrospect."

(Robert Louis Stevenson)

When we put our minds to something

Let's look at a somewhat similar need for action in American science in the not so distant past of our nation's history.

The significance of the following example relates to the power of focused coordinated cooperative scientific action and not the particular resultant scientific accomplishment. I am not trying to suggest that the making of the first atomic weapon was a wonderful human event, but it was an amazing scientific accomplishment which illustrates a scientific research process of great importance to the future of stem cell medicine.

During World War II President Franklin Roosevelt received an urgent communication from Dr. Albert Einstein informing him of a new scientific breakthrough, a new discovery of nature in atomic physics that was destined to change the world forever.

The naturally occurring process was called nuclear fission, whereby under laboratory conditions it was found that if a particular atomic isotope of uranium is bombarded with neutron "bullets," some of the uranium atoms split into halves, releasing nuclear energy by way of Einstein's famous discovery, $E=mc^2$. This natural atom splitting process was found to also "shoot" two additional neutron bullets during each atomic split. It was theorized that the neutron bullets shot out during the uranium atomic splitting process might, under the right conditions, collide with adjacent uranium atoms causing them to also split, yielding more nuclear mass-to-energy conversion and, of course, the production of more neutron bullets, which could theoretically start the process over again in a chain reaction producing an unfathomable burst of nuclear energy release . . . a nuclear bomb.

At the time of Einstein's letter to Roosevelt the only thing separating science from creating an atom splitting bomb was that the particular isotope of uranium required for the chain reaction to occur was found in nature mixed among other more stable atomic isotopes of uranium.

The bomb would be possible only if the bomb-friendly isotope could be purified by isolating it from the vastly more abundant chain reaction unfriendly isotopes in a process called enrichment, a very difficult physics-engineering feat.

Einstein informed Roosevelt that physicists were already working on the enrichment of uranium in Germany for Adolf Hitler at the time of the letter.

The age of nuclear power and the potential for nuclear weapons was foisted upon the planet due to a discovery of nature which was understood by only a handful of scientists in the world.

The news was important—a major shift in world thinking and technology was about to occur. Millions of lives would be affected when someone was able to develop the technology. Both sides knew the basics, and the possibilities, but it would require development of a practical application to change the path of history.

If the U.S. brought all of its resources to bear on development, it could utilize the technology to end the wars it was fighting with forces that sought to enslave the world, save many millions of lives in the process and restore democracy to Europe and other parts of the earth.

Einstein's communication to Roosevelt led to a U.S. government endeavor, the Manhattan Project, which gathered thousands of scientists to work cooperatively, leveraging their efforts by pooling their research. This unprecedented method, the massive pooling of scientific thinking and research, led to an exponentially more effective system of development of this scientific technology.

The discovery of how natural nuclear energy is released changed the world forever—but not until the government sanctioned and funded a broad research effort. The government's involvement was necessary not only because of the destructive capacities of the new technology, but also because of the problem that it was really outside of the normal operating methodologies of investors and developers, just as using Healing Cells are now.

The Manhattan Project achieved a rapid tipping point of consciousness of the new discovery of natural nuclear fission and its implications which created a new scientific research focus. The project cost the U.S. government approximately 30 billion in today's dollars, and employed 6,000 scientists and 134,000 support personnel under the scientific leadership of Dr. Oppenheimer and the military guidance of General Groves. The project was completed under President Truman and lead to the abrupt end of World War II, saving many lives and ending inhumane hardships imposed by sadistic regimes.

Now the world has harnessed the "green" energy of nuclear power to electrify its cities and industries with relative safety.

While I'm no Einstein, or even a Jenner or Fleming, when compared with the natural discoveries of nuclear fission, vaccines or antibiotics, the scientific discovery upon which this book is based, the 2000-DOCS discovery of the human healing organ system, is more important, not less important, than any of these great discoveries of nature as related to the future health and wellbeing of mankind.

This is precisely why we need a Healing Cells "Manhattan Project," a government-private industry partnership project with the aim of developing the most profound medical scientific discovery of the new century which will change the course of human history on the same scale as Dr. Jenner's discovery of the immune system in the early 19th Century and Sir Alexander Fleming's discovery of antibiotics in the beginning of the 20th Century.

President Roosevelt started the Manhattan Project to make a nuclear weapon before Hitler could do so. Adolph Hitler was the common nemesis of that time. Today the enemy is outdated healthcare methodologies which have and continue to abnormally consume our national budget, in extremis, while Americans are becoming the least healthy country in the world (we are 73rd).

The Manhattan Project's stellar success was dependent as much on the cooperation and coordinated sharing and dispersal of information by the 6,000 scientists involved under the guidance and coordination of Dr. Oppenheimer as it was dependent on the amount of money spent for it. The project is emblematic of the principles of coordination, information sharing and scientific focus because it was begun with nothing more than a theory, understood by a handful of individuals around the world that a nuclear energy producing chain reaction might occur if certain conditions could be created (specific isotope sequestration, enrichment), conditions never achieved before Einstein's letter to the President.

This was nothing more than a theory, a notion, an idea, a meme. Scientists together focused on the idea that a chain reaction would occur if the right conditions could be met. And the chain reaction did occur once those theoretical conditions were achieved in real time.

They focused on achieving those conditions, and the theory became reality.

The power of this idea was released through the "magic" of cooperative focus. The Manhattan Project brought together the cooperative efforts of over 6,000 scientists in order to focus on this one thing.

In like manner and for similar reasons, the President and Congress must properly consider this same coordinated focus of the Manhattan Project as a most relevant lesson of U.S. scientific history, which teaches us the unparalleled importance of coordinated focus in scientific research, a factor which cannot be overstated as it is particularly relevant to American Healing Cells therapy research.

If doctors shared their clinical effects, as they happen in a real time outcomes-data system, openly, in a cooperative intelligent team effort as they did in the Manhattan Project, then remarkable results will develop very quickly, without the need for the exorbitant expenses of the drug-molecular formulated methodologies of double blind placebo-controlled research which is undoable for a natural unpatentable therapeutics on the extreme complexity of adult stem cells.

Risk vs. benefit considerations

The risk/benefit issue can often be formidable in medicine and government alike, but sometimes it can be straightforward and even easy, as in a need for surgery to avert a clear and present danger to life or limb. Under "conditions in extremis" within medicine and government alike, the risk-to-benefit equation may demand a dangerous intervention such as surgery for severe chest trauma or in government such as entering World War II because of an attack on the American fleet at Pearl Harbor.

In medicine, and I believe in government, there is also another type of situation in which the risk/benefit analysis demands quick action: specifically, when the risk of intervention is very small and the potential benefits are very great, in which case the intervention is clearly appropriate—an easy decision.

We need a government-private industry partnership project within our current clinical-medical infrastructure that inexpensively will result in a quickly delivered, enduring benefit using a method that does not expand the national budget. A Healing Cells project has enormous potential to benefit our entire society while setting no undesirable precedents. It is an idea for action with an extraordinarily favorable risk-to-benefit ratio. These common sense risk/benefit requirements are fulfilled by the Healing Cells "Manhattan Project" as proposed in this work. It is an example of government action with little or no risk while delivering a potentially enormous and enduring national and international benefit, gargantuan in health benefits and cost reduction. What a superb gift to the people of America and to the world!

Moreover, in the case of the first phase of the Healing Cells project, the cost would be less than minimal. If the FDA would simply lift its unwise and medically unjustified ban on using a patient's own Healing Cells (autologous cell therapeutics) by our nation's doctors, then a paradigm shift in medicine would be triggered automatically at very little cost. The American people would be the beneficiaries of the new Healing Cells therapies, which would rapidly become available quite automatically.

This one quintessentially appropriate government action (to withdraw the FDA ban) would trigger the commencement of immediate and informative direct experience in prescribing a patient's own (autologous) Healing Cells by thousands of our American doctors who would be allowed to prescribe Healing

Cells as long as the clinical results are sent to a data collection site, open to public use and reporting (of course, only patient profiles and treatment descriptions are necessary, not patient identities). The rest would be automatic.

Unless the medical lobby in Washington politically crushes such an idea - after all, those who profit from the status quo can be expected to do everything in their power to stop this health windfall from getting to the people who need it most.

As it stands now, Healing Cells are obviously destined to be the "better mouse trap." Is it un-American to keep this better mouse trap out of the competition in our American market? If the Healing Cells ban is lifted, the American public will become healthier and wealthier. Not a bad outcome, available and doable with minimal risk.

I don't know what they call this kind of decision in government, but in medicine we call it "a no-brainer."

The FDA is changing the course of medical history in the wrong direction, due either to ignorance or corruption.

We need the Healing Cells "Manhattan Project" because our current research system does not provide the necessary pathway of coordinated scientific focus in an information-sharing intellectual environment, which will be required for our country to reach the next step in the evolution of human medicine, the Healing Cells therapeutic paradigm.

Phase One: retraction of the FDA's ban on using a patient's own (autologous) Healing Cells

While there is some research in using a patient's own Healing Cells for therapy (an autologous transplantation) occurring in some medical centers in the U.S., they are puny studies that are entirely insufficient and unsophisticated given the monumental importance of these cells to the development of a science which is destined to solve our country's wellbeing and healthcare cost crisis.

Clinical and laboratory experience with a patient's own Healing Cells (autologous) are an indispensable first step for science to investigate Healing Cells treatment, in general because when these cells heal the human body, the processes involve safe but complex biological mechanisms that we have yet to fully and properly understand. We know that treatment works and that it will benefit the patient, but we need to collect data to tell us when to treat, how often, and with which particular types of Healing Cells to maximize the benefits to the patient and minimize the cost of treatment.

The art and science of medicine have advanced through history only through meticulous study of nature which provides the understanding required to imitate nature in the development of new derivative therapies. We cannot imitate nature unless and until we focus on the lessons that nature has to teach us. Doctors and medical scientists must intensely study Healing Cells obtained from the patient's own (autologous) body clinically and in the laboratory to unlock nature's secrets of human cellular healing. Certainly this must happen first, before trying to improve upon nature with inventions. Intense coordinated focus is how human medicine always advances—this is the lesson of history.

The only two previous huge medical evolutionary events in memory, the development of antibiotics and vaccines, teach us that the big discovery yields no benefit to society until and unless science changes its focus to the discovery, a difficult cultural process.

Roger M. Nocera, M.D.

Penicillin, the natural fungus, was studied intensely to learn how it killed bacteria. Once we learned penicillin's natural anti-bacterial bio-molecular code (bio-chemical interference with bacterial wall development during reproduction) we were able to harness it, and only then to imitate it. Soon we were inventing derivative molecular antibiotics that could destroy every type of bacteria, not just the few that penicillin could kill. Man trumped nature by learning from her first. We focused research on nature until nature yielded her secrets; that is the only way that medical science truly advances.

The same pattern of human advancement occurred after the discovery of the immune system. Our doctors and medical scientists studied how the immune system worked in clinics and laboratories. Yet vaccines were produced and saved lives long before the scientific details concerning the natural immune system's biological activities were fully understood. That is why Jenner was such a genius; he destroyed disease and saved lives even though he actually knew a small amount of valid information about the human immune organ system. But what Jenner knew was right to accomplish a quantum leap in medicine for humanity because great genius is never measured in amount of knowledge, rather, quality of knowledge—in this case critical and pivotal knowledge about the human immune system. Focus.

The immune system remains under intense scientific investigation today. Vaccines of all types were developed over the decades as we studied and learned how our immune system actually works. This appropriate level of humility and reverence for nature is a minimal requirement for great advancements in the art and science of medicine.

We must now intensely focus research on patients' own (autologous) Healing Cells' biological healing activities because we have only begun to understand how they heal our bodies. This focus will teach doctors how healing, particularly cellular healing, occurs in the human body so that we may augment its effects as we have with every prior pivotal discovery of nature.

We all have huge supplies of extra Healing Cells

Autologous Healing Cells are perfectly safe because they are cells taken out of one part of the body and simply put back into another body part of the same patient. Clearly, taking Healing Cells from the same person that will be treated with them is going to be readily accepted by both patients and doctors because of the obvious benign nature of this therapy, notwithstanding the medical incorrectness of the current FDA ban on the use of these cells.

So, how and why do autologous Healing Cells work so well?

Throughout life, as we have been saying, the Healing Cells within bone marrow are triggered hormonally to reproduce and increase in number by cytokines released from injured tissue cells.

Healing Cells increase in the blood and then are attracted to the injured tissue by the cytokine mediated process of chemo-attraction, whereby they heal the body exactly where the damage is located: targeted cellular healing. For some reason, many of these Healing Cells become trapped within fat tissue and are never again available to help heal the body. Trillions of healthy Healing Cells become trapped inside our body fat tissue starting from a very early age where they stay in a quiet metabolic state for years and years, without being available to the bloodstream for delivery to injured tissue. Because the Healing Cells are inactive while they reside in fat tissue, they do not reproduce or otherwise function, which keeps them young compared with the rest of the body because reproduction and activity of cells ages them by wear and tear of functioning and the shortening of their DNA telomeres.

Medical scientists have learned to extract these valuable Healing Cells from fat by liposuction. Once these cells are collected, a connective tissue dissolving enzyme is introduced into the fatty fluid to release the Healing Cells from their sleepy fat tissue trap. These valuable Healing Cells are then simply re-injected safely back into the patient, where they are free to perform their amazing natural healing activities. The procedure is entirely safe and quite effective as it involves nothing more than releasing a patient's own Healing Cells into a different body compartment where they are free to perform their natural healing functions because they are no longer trapped in the fat compartment where they are unavailable to heal.

Moreover, although they are not legal to use in the U.S. according to the FDA, their use is perfectly safe, and one cannot even imagine how harm could befall a patient simply because cells are transplanted from one part of the body to another.[45, 46, 47, 48, 49, 50, 51, 52, 53, 56, 57, 58, 59, 60, 61, 62, 63, 64] Skin grafts and lip plumps are similar autologous tissue transplantations, which are likewise perfectly safe and have been legal in the U.S. for decades.

At our overseas clinics we have treated rheumatoid arthritis and multiple sclerosis using fat derived autologous Healing Cells treatments with consistent and monumental success without a single adverse complication of any kind. Yet the FDA will not allow your doctor to prescribe this simple autologous tissue graft technique in our country outside of expensive and highly restricted, puny and unsophisticated FDA approved clinical research trials, because autologous Healing Cells are impossible to patent, and therefore very little funding for these trials is available, resulting in the dearth of these important clinical experiences.

Pharmaceutical drugs approved by the FDA for treatment of rheumatoid arthritis and multiple sclerosis have many serious side effects and are exorbitantly expensive (tens of thousands a year), yet they are not only legal but also de facto required, while transferring one's own Healing Cells, which has no adverse side effects and is extremely effective, remains illegal by the FDA.

Why? As a physician I absolutely do not know why this obstructive medical regulation exists. But I do know to a medical certainty that this problem must be resolved if we are ever to advance medical therapeutics to the next evolutionary phase, which is now at the world's medical doorstep, knocking, unanswered.

Tracking our progress
There is an old technique for tracing white blood cells in nuclear medicine imaging used to detect the site of infection in a patient with fever of unknown origin (FUO) called an abscess scan[65], which was very important before it was supplanted by the invention of cross sectional imaging in which the infection process could be directly imaged and diagnosed with precision.

In this largely obsolete nuclear medicine test, a patient who is suspected of harboring an infection somewhere in her body has a small amount of blood drawn, which is spun down in a centrifuge so that the white blood cells float to the top (the Buffy-coat). Some of the patient's white blood cells are thusly obtained and tagged with a safe medical radio tracer called 99m Technetium. Once tagged with Technetium the white blood cells from the buffy-coat are injected back into the patient, a tiny autologous transplantation. Then these radio tracer-labeled white blood cells do what white blood cells do, which is to be attracted by cytokines released by infected, injured tissue cells, wherever they may be within the body. The patient is then evaluated with gamma camera pictures that detect the location of the tagged white blood cells within her body. The diagnostic images reveal the site of infection or abscess, where the radio tracer tagged white blood cells accumulate.

The same type of procedure is easily adapted to Healing Cells treatments so that Healing Cells clinics can easily radio-tracer tag with a 99m Technetium kit, like those found in any nuclear medicine department in the country, about 10 percent of the Healing Cells to be injected into the same patient that they came from (autologous). The resultant diagnostic gamma-camera images taken after injection of the cells will readily demonstrate the tagged Healing Cells' exact locations within the patient's body, which will establish whether the Healing Cells have "homed" to the injured tissues (by chemotaxis). These special medical pictures detect the physiological performance of the Healing Cells protocols selected for treatment in the individual patient and her disease.

This is critical prognostic information because we know that Healing Cells will heal only if they "home" to injured tissues first (cytokine specific chemo-attraction). "Failure to home" is the greatest clinical obstacle to successful Healing Cells treatments of any kind, and will continue to be the greatest obstacle for decades to come in Healing Cells medicine. The Healing cells "Manhattan Project" should provide us with the desperately needed data to help us assist this homing process. Homing diagnostic medical imaging of Healing Cells is an important, clinically obtainable, objective determinate of Healing Cells treatment success. This easily obtainable clinical information will accelerate our understanding of Healing Cells medicine rapidly. Our experience overseas has taught us that knowing when we have given enough Healing Cells and the correct type of Healing Cells at the correct time within the disease process are the most challenging aspects of clinical stem cell medicine, but we know these parameters matter a great deal in the success or failure of Healing Cells therapy.

What research is needed?

The most important parameter of Healing Cells treatment protocols is the timing of a Healing Cells injection because success relates to the stage of the individual patient's disease process (patho-physiologic stage). This aspect of the treatment is the most complicated because of the enormous number of possible permutations of clinically important timing variables of Healing Cells administration.

For example, if the disease is within an inactive stage (non-inflammatory phase of its pathogenesis) then Healing Cells will not home to the site of tissue injury. Healing Cells require active cell injury to create the special hormone-like signal (cytokines released by injured cells) for the attraction and cell homing process to occur (cytokine, tissue specific chemo-attraction). All disease processes have widely variable and only partly understood hormonal (cytokine) signal dynamics, which are usually complicated and often multi-phased. Only massive direct clinical experience with Healing Cells treatments using objective data analysis, such as nuclear medicine tracer labeled Healing Cells homing studies, will provide the treatment regimen information that is lacking. This information will be needed to develop the best protocol "recipes" of how many and what type and in what order Healing Cells should be given for each disease, customized for each individual patient to be treated. In other words, they will provide us with the "standard of care" for each disease being treated with Healing Cells. This is the destiny of medical practice all over the world for the next century, which will change the world and the human condition on this planet forever.

This is the best pathway available to efficiently acquire the massive information that will be required to develop a successful Healing Cells therapeutic paradigm. It would not be long before Healing Cells' diagnostic "homing images" will guide all clinical use of Healing Cells treatments for each and every disease in each individual patient. Just one quick example may make the point clear.

Mesenchymal Healing Cells are tremendously anti-inflammatory. If a disease required them for treatment, as well as, say, CD+34 Healing Cells, then the powerfully anti-inflammatory mesenchymal Healing Cells should be given last, as they tend to decrease the cytokine production of inflammatory cytokines which are part of the inflammatory process that mesenchymal Healing Cells turn off (down regulate). But if given first this also turns off the chemo-attraction cytokine signal needed for homing of the CD+34 Healing Cells to the site of cell injury. Of course, homing nuclear tracer studies will reveal if this is an issue in any given situation. If the CD+34 healing cells home to the injury site in large enough numbers, which is proportional to the nuclear tracer counts and is therefore measurable, then the treatment will be a success, but if they do not home to the site of injury, healing will not take place properly.

This approach of learning as you go, safely, will work by shortening the road to successful Healing Cells treatments such that it would not be long before many old invasive, painful, unnatural, high-tech medical paradigm therapies will become obsolete, dying as they should in an unceremonious, gradual decline as the new therapeutic paradigm of Healing Cells begins to emerge and demonstrate better results that are less expensive in clinics all over the U.S.

The Healing Cells "Manhattan Project" – Phase One, will remove the illogical FDA ban on a doctor's right to use a patient's own (autologous) Healing Cells. We would thereby set free our nation's doctors to use their medical educations in combination with these healing cells in American clinics. Homing diagnostic imaging will help determine best practice protocols for each disease process, advancing this science very quickly. The Healing Cells "Manhattan Project" would set up a required data center, whereby ordinary doctors can add Healing Cells to their treatment protocols, but they must report the results to the Healing Cells research analysis team. Analysis of this kind of data would rapidly advance our knowledge of the efficacy of different Healing Cells protocols, which could be published so that every doctor's clinical experiences with them would be pooled, shared feely and updated.

Doctors will more profoundly enjoy the practice of medicine again, inasmuch as practicing the routine American standard of care medicine is rather unfulfilling and robotic to persons who have dedicated over 10 years of college education and much of their lives to healing, yet have been caught in a system that forces them to follow the same old pathways of unnatural (and even dangerous) standard of care therapeutics, which has become so ineffectual and crude that the joy of practicing medicine has become all but non-existent for many doctors.

Doctors would not have to learn to become cell biologists, just as I did not have to become a magnet physicist in order to interpret MRI images from our magnet. There are PhDs for that. All doctors must do is prescribe a Healing Cells treatment on a prescription pad. There will be plenty of technical support and information flowing within the same infrastructure that we have now, except there will be lab technicians to process the cells, ready to be prescribed. Doctors must be given their civil and medical freedom to choose the best treatments for their patients according to their high level of medical education and clinical judgment. Doctors could tap their creativity and medical analytic prowess as they once could before medicine became so fixed in recipe "standard of care" medicine.

Our overly unnatural, high-tech and exorbitantly expensive therapies will die a natural death because the statistics for successful treatments with patients' own Healing Cells (autologous) will be disseminated to doctors and patients alike, which will trigger a demand for these natural treatments because they will be more successful in healing diseases than our current unnatural 10 percent cure rate high tech treatments.

Phase Two: lifting the ban on afterbirth-derived allogeneic Healing Cells

Afterbirth derived (allogeneic) Healing Cells are illegal to use in American clinics, yet not a single one of the over 500 patients treated at our overseas clinics has had any significant side effects from these cells. Healing Cells derived from the afterbirth of normal pregnancies are illegal in the U.S. only because the FDA designates them so, not because they are harmful in any way medically.[66, 67, 68, 69, 70, 71, 72, 73, 74, 75, 76, 77, 78, 79, 80, 81, 82] This is true, whether it is well known or not. The old ways are artificially perpetuated by investors that want to patent stem cells by manufacturing them with their patentable technology from Embryonic Building Stem Cells, either natural or manmade. Our government leaders and citizens must understand that this costly maneuver is nothing more than an unnecessary scheme perpetrated for the purpose of profiteering on the backs of our country's ill patients, our loved ones.

"Repetition does not transform a lie into a truth."

(Franklin D. Roosevelt)

The FDA claims that afterbirth (allogeneic) Healing Cells need to be proven safe before they can approve them for use (lift their ban on doctors' freedom to prescribe them). Did you know that these same cells (allogeneic from cord blood derived CD+34 cells) have been used legally since 1984 in the U.S. for one purpose that is exempt from the FDA ban? These cells can be legally used for bone marrow replacement for cancer patients who have had their bone marrow obliterated with cancer chemotherapy and radiation therapy.[83, 84, 85, 86, 87, 88, 89, 90] Hundreds of thousands of patients have been treated successfully in the U.S. using these Healing Cells from afterbirth from normal, healthy deliveries to reestablish bone marrow. Yet for any other clinical use these cells are illegal in the U.S.

Is this logical?

Is this rational medical thinking?

If you ask your doctor about this he may tell you that those bone marrow replacement treatments cause autoimmune disease. That is true. But it is not true using methodologies we use to treat patients overseas. Here is why.

The few doctors in the U.S. who have been involved with afterbirth-derived allogeneic Healing Cells (CD+34 cord blood derived allogeneic hematopoietic regeneration) for bone marrow replacement do not understand that it is the absence of a functioning bone marrow immune system that causes the autoimmune disease side effect in these patients. U.S. doctors usually do not know that autoimmune disease does not occur when allogeneic Healing Cells are given to patients who have an intact bone marrow; they never have that clinical situation in their work because U.S. doctors are banned from giving these cells to anyone who has an intact bone marrow.[90]

The chemotherapy which is used to kill the cancer cells also wipes out the bone marrow cells. The cancer treatment kills the patient's bone marrow, which is why they need the allogeneic Healing Cells in the first place. Since the effector-cells of the immune system reside within the bone marrow they too are killed with the cancer treatment. When the afterbirth derived allogeneic Healing Cells are given to these patients, the tissue vacuum in the immune system is taken up by a new immune system, which is developed by the transplanted allogeneic Healing Cells. This new immune system does not recognize the patient's body as self. Therefore, the new immune system created by the allogeneic Healing Cells attacks the patient's body tissues in a disease called autoimmunity. What most American doctors working with allogeneic Healing Cells for bone marrow replacement don't understand is that if these allogeneic Healing Cells are given to a patient who has an intact bone marrow, the stem cells do not have a vacuum to fill, so no new bone marrow immune system is created and therefore, auto-immune disease never develops in these patients.

Because American doctors only work with afterbirth-derived Healing Cells in bone marrow depleted patients and never with patients who have intact bone marrow immune systems, they remain unaware of the safety of allogeneic Healing Cells (cord blood derived adult stem cells, CD34+ cells) when used for purposes other than bone marrow replacement. They erroneously conclude that autoimmune complications occur with afterbirth allogeneic Healing Cells transplantations. Yet patients with intact bone marrow do not experience auto-immune diseases—ever, which is why we give Healing Cells in overseas clinics without immune suppressive drugs of any kind and we don't see any side effects, autoimmune or otherwise.

The fact that all mothers have all their children's Healing Cells in their bone marrow for life, and all their babies have cells living in mother's body for life, for example inside mother's brain, liver, heart, etc. (maternal microchimerism) is further proof that afterbirth derived allogeneic Healing Cells are safe and natural.[91, 92, 93, 94, 95, 96, 97, 98, 99, 100, 101, 102] All mothers benefit from this allogeneic transplantation from their children during pregnancy, as suggested by the direct relationship between maternal longevity and the number of live births mothers experience as well as the evidence that a pregnant mother with hepatitis during pregnancy will have many more of her child's cells occupying and functioning inside her liver after a pregnancy in this clinical setting. Some have contended that mothers can get autoimmunity from maternal microchimerism, yet that has since been largely proven incorrect.[103]

Also, patients who have received a whole blood transfusion also receive the Healing Cells that are always in the blood. This is a safe allogeneic Healing Cells transplantation as well, albeit a small one. Not so small are the umbilical cord blood transfusions, rich in Healing Cells that have been reported in the peer review literature.[66, 67, 68, 69, 70, 71, 72, 73, 74, 75, 76, 77, 78, 79, 80, 81, 82] As reported in Lancet in a study from India where umbilical cord blood rich in allogeneic Healing Cells was used to treat anemia patients during blood shortages in malaria epidemics, it was demonstrated that no adverse side effects from this large infusion of allogeneic Healing Cells ever occurred. Over 400 units of umbilical cord blood rich in Healing Cells were given without complication in the Lancet report.

The second important step after the removal of the FDA ban on autologous Healing Cells will be to fund research with allogeneic afterbirth-derived Healing Cells that will be required to undo the medically unjustified FDA ban on these cells as well.

In our current research system, medical doctors are the only citizens actually trained to know which therapeutic research focus will be best medically for our citizens, but they are never in position to decide it. These decisions are exclusively made by non-medical business people who control the hundreds of millions of dollars needed for proof of efficacy medical research of any significance. These enormously expensive decisions are based on profitability, largely a matter of patentability, and strategies to obtain market share within the future stem cell therapeutic space. The best financial result for those investors who currently control medical research would be a huge delay in the development of any Healing Cells therapeutics, as they could never be more profitable for them than the current synthetic drug-based therapeutic American medical paradigm, especially now that the baby boomers are in their medical care consumer age.

The original Manhattan Project cost approximately 30 billion in today's dollars, which is a pittance compared with the 2,400 billion (2.4 trillion) dollars spent each year on medical care in the U.S. Moreover, simply redacting the medically illogical FDA ban on a patient's own (autologous) Healing Cells treatments by our nation's doctors would trigger the rapid acquisition of critical clinical information, whereby Healing Cells therapy protocols could be developed rapidly, cheaply, safely and effectively, without the cost prohibitive need to do extensive proof of efficacy research.

CHAPTER SEVEN

MEDICAL CREDENTIALS

"My doctor is nice; every time I see him,

I'm ashamed of what I think of doctors in general."

(McLaughlin)

MY MEDICAL CREDENTIALS?

A fair question.

My formal professional medical credentials and formal medical and science education are an appropriate and healthy topic of this book. I hope that your intelligence makes you reluctant to accept at face value the medical scientific opinions in his book on so profoundly important a national medical issue as stem cells without some strong reason to believe me.

The computer Information age

We suffer collectively from a disconnection to valid information in the U.S. today. Ironically, we suffer from a disconnection to valid information exactly because we are so far into the modern information age, spawned largely by the computer age. This ailment affects every part of our modern human life.

We are suffering from maladjustment to the constant mountains of information constantly being thrown at us in our culture within new information channels of hypermodern and untested advanced technology being served up to us in every conceivable category of our lives in formats and methodologies foreign to our common historical.

The information age problem is nothing more than being exposed on a continual basis in real time to more and more information at an ever increasing pace than we are able to digest adequately—more information than we can possibly deal with effectively in its entirety.

Our information age is actually much like the first year of medical school, as I recall.

We start in medical school knowing that we could never learn what is already known medically about the human heart even if we studied for a decade, and more medical details about the human heart become known every year.

This is true as well for the central nervous system, the gastrointestinal system, the pulmonary, renal, skeletal, urogenital, endocrine, hematopoietic, vascular systems, etc. So the medical school professors start to throw medical information out at medical students in a frenzy beginning on day one. It never stops, ever, not for four years of medical school, not for the years spent in teaching hospital residency and not really even after 30 years of learning and practicing medicine, because the medical information age has been blasting out medical information at an exponential clip for decades.

The key to dealing with too much information, as every doctor knows, is selective learning.

Medical doctors of today are as good, no more and no less, than the success they achieved in answering this question for as long as they have been doctors … **what is important to know in medicine about anything and everything available to know?**

Lord knows we can't learn all of it.

It's a continuing question to every doctor every minute that they are medical doctors. It's a question that no one can or does answer perfectly, nor do many answer it perfectly wrongly either, and still survive in the profession. But we must continuously answer this question, hopefully not by default, but rather with growing medical wisdom as we proceed through our long medical careers. While all information has its place, we can't give information a place in our heads at the rate that it comes at us now so we must choose, even if god-forbid we choose by default because we don't consciously and competently choose wisely.

My medical education formally began with undergraduate degrees in premed undergraduate biological sciences and chemistry. All premed students at that time who would eventually matriculate to major university medical schools in America were expected to take the hardest premed courses and expected to earn nearly all A's in every course, which if achieved automatically inducted us into the national academic honor societies of Phi Beta Kappa and Phi Kappa Phi upon graduation. Here is a partial list of those pre-med courses: genetics, cell biology, biochemistry, physiology, comparative anatomy, zoology, botany, inorganic chemistry, advanced differential and integral calculus, ecology, epidemiology, atomic physics, general physics and quantum physics.

I arrived at the University of Massachusetts Medical School, which was filled with other nearly all "A"- earning cream of the crop-type medical students who graduated with similar national honors from the local undergraduate New England universities like MIT, Harvard, Princeton, Tufts, Yale, Brandies, BU and BC. We dissected our cadavers together in human anatomy, learned the most advanced medical science from world-class medical scientists, mostly from ivory tower New England Universities, in courses like human biochemistry, physiology, cell biology, general histology, human gross and microscopic pathology, histopathology, cytopathology, human genetics, pharmacology, infectious diseases, immunology, neurology and neuropathology, to name a few.

Then the most amazing thing that ever happened to me in my life happened — the rubber hit the road with a vengeance.

All of a sudden, all those medical students started their 3rd year of medical school, the clinical years in the major local New England hospitals whereupon our nervous breakdowns started to worsen. We thought important medical information could not be thrown at us any faster than those first 2 years of medical school. We were wrong.

In that moment we had crossed into a totally new paradigm, aptly called the real world of clinical hospital medicine.

This is a life and death place.

Our academic theories about medicine hit reality on a grand scale, head-on at a speed of well over a hundred miles an hour. A constant diet of important medical information now was coming at us in public in a highly sophisticated and technical world at the core of medical and surgical activities concerning grave trauma and other grave illnesses in a very real world.

We were constantly diagnosing, triaging, treating, hurting, helping, doing progressively more important and dangerous medical and surgical procedures, getting it right, getting it wrong, correcting fast and moving on, always moving on to another whole world of its own like cardiology, pediatrics, obstetrics, neonatology, pediatric surgery, trauma surgery, orthopedics, gynecology, emergency medicine, general medicine, neurosurgery, oncology, code team duty (often 4-5 codes per day), gastroenterology, diagnostic imaging, cardiac surgery, rheumatology, plastic surgery, pain medicine, infectious diseases, pulmonology, thoracic surgery, endocrinology, pathology, histology, hematology, dermatology and psychiatry.

It was like an explosion going off in our heads.

The problem with this world is that until you know its ins and outs, the amount of new important medical information that comes your way as a medical student and young doctor is beyond comprehension, a comprehension that ultimately takes a decade at least to develop adequately in most major American medical specialties.

That 3rd year of medical school at Worchester City Hospital and U-Mass Medical Center I found myself falling in love with that crazy hospital world filled to the brim with severe real life drama. This world was reality, plus; a complex, multifactorial human and technical reality paradigm on steroids.

I have spent 30 years in that major hospital world, two years at the teaching hospitals of U-Mass Medical Center and five years at the famous and enormous John Sealy Teaching Hospital and Shrine Burn Center of the University of Texas Medical School in Galveston, a fellowship period at the likewise famous Arms Forces Institute of Pathology in Washington, D.C., and the next 17 years in mostly major Trauma I-level Hospitals in the Phoenix metropolitan area.

There are a few interesting historical intersections of major industries and my medical specialty of diagnostic medical imaging that will help you to understand my medical perspective, which is, of course, ubiquitous in this book.

It really all started with advances in physics, especially atomic physics in the earlier 20th Century. In fact, my specialty has two trunks of its tree. Conrad Roentgen, the grandfather of my specialty, discovered x-rays with his subatomic particle cathode ray tube and later the first x-ray picture of a hand. Atomic physics also focused on natural radiation, which created nuclear energy science and nuclear medical science, which is a fascinating innovative medical diagnostic and therapeutic tool using natural radiation from natural radioactive isotopes used for organ metabolic imaging tests and radiation therapy for cancer.

Positron emission tomography (PET) is likewise an extension of nuclear physics and bio-medical applications using positron natural radiation and cross sectional advanced 3-dimentional Fourier mathematical analysis. Since much of nuclear medicine involves diagnostic medical imaging, my specialty has always strongly dominated the field. We use radiation to treat hyperthyroidism with radioactive iodine, I133, cobalt for cancer, etc. These two limbs of diagnostics had already developed much of my specialty of radiology, or diagnostic imaging, before I started in the specialty.

Once the computer revolution started it triggered a paradigm shift in all of hospital and clinical medicine, which just started in medicine about three decades ago when I entered my specialty of medical and surgical diagnostics.

The computer revolution spawned the invention of computerized axial tomography (CAT scans) and real time ultrasound imaging, which both use revolutionary advanced calculus called Fourier-mathematics to detect then reconstruct with computer aid and massive computation speed the 3-D space images within a patient's body. It is called collectively cross sectional imaging and it revolutionized all of medicine in at least one major way in every specialty, but more often it revolutionized much of each medical and surgical specialty in many ways.

Because diagnostic cross sectional imaging demonstrates each and every body part so elegantly it has literally revolutionized every other specialty diagnostically and often therapeutically within virtually all of modern medicine over the past three decades.

Diagnostic life-and-death medical and surgical decisions are now routinely made using the most sophisticated diagnostic equipment known to mankind, in the specialty I have engaged for nearly three decades.

After it all began we soon were looking at pregnant women's unborn babies' lips to see a cleft palate, unborn babies' spines to see damage that would cripple the child for life, to see a double bubble-sign of duodenal atresia or a fetal tiny heart (hypo-plastic left heart syndrome or a Tetralogy of Fallot), or water on the brain (hydrocephalus) so treatment will be available emergently when these children are born with these, and many more detectable diseases.

We saw twins, conjoined twins, potentially fatal placenta positions (placenta-previa and placental-abruption), potentially fatal ectopic pregnancies, pregnancy cancers (chorio-carcinoma), anencephaly, spina-bifida, Turner's syndrome, erythroblastosis-fetalis, fetal ascites, atresias, etc., now for the first time with ultrasound cross sectional medical imaging.

In other patients with CAT scans and ultrasound cross sectional imaging we could now find things better than any tapping on the back of a patient with a doctors finger or listening with his stethoscope—for example: a lung cancer, a deadly blood vessel rupture (a dissecting aortic aneurysm) or uterine cancer in the elderly, ovarian cancer in young women, pancreatic cancer, brain tumors, carotid stenosis ready to produce a fatal stroke (cerebral infarcts from thrombo-emboli), brain bleeding (idiopathic, traumatic, AVM or berry aneurisms), blood clots in leg veins that can lead to sudden death from pulmonary thrombo-emboli, brain clots (sinus thrombosis), water on the brain (obstructive and non-obstructive hydrocephalus), head and neck tumors (parotid, salivary, nose and throat cancers), eye tumors, eye socket disease (orbital fractures, cancers, Graves thyroid disease), all lung diseases like lung cancer, COPD, lung infections, tuberculosis, coccidiodalmycosis, sarcoidosis, mesotheliomas. Also we could now see appendicitis, diverticulitis, hiatal hernias, ruptured bowel, ischemic bowel, liver and gall bladder diseases (hepatitis, abscess, cholocystitis, biliary obstructions, hepatoma, cholangiocarcinoma, portal hypertension and cirrhosis, etc., etc.), abdominal aortic aneurysms, aortic dissections, abnormalities in heart wall thickness, heart wall motion (kinetics), heart infarcts and ischemia, all orthopedics (bone neoplastic disease, multiple myeloma, meniscal tears, rotator cuff injuries and all other internal derangements, etc, etc.) . This and so much more those in the specialty of diagnostic medical imaging science must master, unequivocally.

My particular medical specialty quite serendipitously happens to have become a major player in all serious illnesses and also in all severe trauma and in every other specialty working in all major hospitals in America over the last three decades.

A cardiologist focuses on the heart, a pulmonologist on lungs, an oncologist on tumors, etc. Unavoidably and unfortunately, most modern day medical specialists know more and more about less and less.

Einstein himself was very aware of this effect of narrowed perspective that scientific specialization engenders when he observed, "Specialization makes it increasingly difficult to keep even our general understanding of science as a whole, without which the true spirit of research is inevitably handicapped . . . Every serious scientific worker is painfully conscious of this involuntary relegation to an ever-narrowing sphere of knowledge, which threatens to deprive the investigator of his broad horizon and degrades him to the level of a mechanic."

Virtually all medical specialties narrow a physician's medical perspective and medical gestalt in order that they focus on the ever growing specific information constantly emerging in ever finer detail in their specialty.

The opposite happens in my specialty of diagnostic imaging because it brings you face to face with virtually every disease and the result of every disease treatment in every medical specialty. This is a critical element of my credentials to write this book because medical specialization in all other instances represents an unfortunate but necessary relegation of a doctor's focus, which unfortunately narrows perspective of medicine as a whole.

A direct kill
There is a gallows-humor term used in some quarters in medicine. The term is "a direct-kill," and it may help to understand how modern diagnostic medical imaging functions today in every major hospital in the country, since the development of cross sectional imaging.

A direct-kill in a hospital community is when the inappropriate action of someone in the hospital, a doctor or a nurse, becomes the primary and immediate cause of a wrongful death of a particular patient in the hospital. A direct-kill is a terrible, terrible occurrence, and it happens easily and quickly in a major metropolitan hospital. The requirement for cooperation, accurate communication and coordinated medical team work is crucial in this stressful world.

The function of "morbidity and mortality rounds" is to educate all hospital departments of past pitfalls which led to past medical misadventures in the hospital that month, like direct kills, god forbid. A "direct kill" can be and often is due to a failure to accurately diagnose something in a timely fashion or due to a failure to perform a clinical duty with proper caution or professional dispatch without impairment or deviation from proper medical practice criteria, which are specialty-specific, memorialized by each specialty-board in volumes of manuals on proper practices in that specialty.

An incompetent and or otherwise impaired neurosurgeon doctor can without a doubt, cause a "direct-kill," but only in patients on the neurosurgery service.

An incompetent or impaired doctor doing my specialty of medical-imaging diagnostics in a major hospital can potentially direct-kill many patients from any and all specialty services because of our central role in all major critical, life and death diagnostic determinations and decisions in all specialties, all day long in every hospital in America and the world.

The medical credentials which I bring to this book involve specialty training in medical image diagnosis including advanced magnetic resonance imaging (MRI), computed axial tomography (CAT scans), diagnostic ultrasound, nuclear medicine, and all other diagnostic medical imaging technology and the understanding which I bring to this book has been informed by a unique clinical experience during my tenure as the chief medical officer and a member of the board of directors for one of the first international Healing Cells biotech companies, an experience unfortunately not available to most doctors today. **Moreover, I have been at the front lines of the paradigm shift over in my specialty as the world changing effects of cross-sectional medical imaging such as CAT scans, MRI, ultrasound, PET, and SECT bourgeoned in America**

Roger M. Nocera, M.D.

over the past three decades in hospital and clinic medical practices.

More recently, I have witnessed the results of over 500 patient treatments with both autologous and allogeneic Healing Cells medical science treatments for many disease processes. I have seen firsthand how sick patients respond to intravenous injections of both autologous and allogeneic Healing Cells and how cell treatment protocols evolve through clinical experience and outcome information feedback.

Quite serendipitously, I have come to all this and also how classic nuclear medical imaging will play a central role in Healing Cells clinical research once it is started in earnest. This unique medical experience has made it eminently clear to me what our future Twenty-First Century medical therapeutic paradigm is destined to look like, how it will develop and the results that can be reasonably anticipated.

Experience in therapeutics in overseas clinics has taught me that the treatments for many diseases would be discovered very rapidly once our doctors focus on natural Healing Cells treatments.

Many of you are not going to like what is said in the next chapter, but the information will help you. When you finish the next chapter you will no longer be a "virgin" about stem cells in America, but you will gain in the needed strength of medical truth and wisdom constantly thereafter.

CHAPTER EIGHT

RELIGION, POLITICS AND STEM CELLS

"I am compelled to fear that science will be used to promote the

power of dominant groups,

rather than to make men happy."

(Bertrand Russell)

Roger M. Nocera, M.D.

America's stem cell cultural disease

To the President of the United States of America, Mr. Obama, for whom I voted . . . twice, once in the primary and again in the general election, and to my fellow pro-science, pro-intellectual liberal Democrats, with all due respect: I wrote this book primarily to help YOU, because I am one of you. You are not going to be pleased to hear what I now have to say about medical embryonic stem cell research. I acutely sense that you are in no mood to be told that you got the medical science screwed-up and just plain wrong about embryonic stem cells, which will become clear in this chapter that I saved purposely for last.

I am not a particularly religious person, nor am I specifically against clinical abortion if reasonable and prudent medically. I do not attend church, synagogue or mosque. I have studied comparative religion and I am personally convinced that the original valid ideas of most modern day religions have not survived intact in modern religious practices. The following quotes by Allan Watts and Albert Einstein confess my actual beliefs as it relates to religion:

> "The common error of ordinary religious practice
> is to mistake the symbol for the reality, to look at
> the finger pointing the way and then to suck it for
> comfort rather than follow it."

> (Alan Watts)

> "What humanity owes to personalities like Budd-
> ha, Moses, and Jesus ranks for me higher than all

the achievements of the enquiring and construc-
tive mind. What these blessed men have given us
we must guard and try to keep alive with all our
strength if humanity is not to lose its dignity, the
security of its existence, and its joy in living."

(Dr. Albert Einstein)

What is to come in this chapter, therefore, is not an anti-abortion
political religious view. Rather it is my medical scientific view,
carefully stated.

My fellow liberal Democratic intellectuals, I know it's going to
be hard to hear that you were tricked by ivory tower stem cell
scientists who let the country and the world down as did their
counterparts in Dr. Jenner's day. But it might help ease the sting
if you admit that you have been following them on stem cells
like some Catholics following the dictates of the Pope in Rome,
without intellectually advanced questioning.

Now, having made that intellectual mistake our country needs
your intellectual clarity, a clarity despoiled by believing lies
about stem cell science from stem cell scientists who are under
the control of a wayward American science industry (as Eisenhower warned).

"In comparing religious belief to science,

I try to remember that science is belief also."

(Vincent de Paul)

It is worrisome that the very people who are most likely to respect good science, have a pro-intellectual and a dispassionate rational approach in their analysis of stem cells and are most likely to be able to read this book and benefit by it are also my fellow liberal Democrats who are highly motivated to not accept the truth that is coming in this chapter because sadly, they have been bamboozled by the ivory tower "experts" on stem cell research, a matter of continuing national relevance, an embarrassing problem for the "pro-science" Democrats.

What happens next in American medicine, without doubt, for good or ill, will affect our loved ones without respect to labels such as republican, independent or democrat.

This book is about medical reality, not politics, and certainly not religion. I anticipate robust attack from opponents (the embryonic stem cell advocates and their financial backers) to my scientific medical views and welcome those medical science challenges with open professional arms.

I do not welcome any accusation that what I am now going to tell you about the embryonic stem cell industry is influenced by religious beliefs, because that would be the opposite of the truth.

I am not anti-abortion and I'm in favor of *Roe v. Wade*.

Please remember, all my fellow liberal intellectuals, it was your ongoing decision to believe these ivory tower experts on stem cells, a little bit like groupies or cult members, as they made you wrong on stem cells by convincing you that only religious zealotry could explain any objection to the validity of embryonic stem cell science, although much of the time you do hear it, it may prove to be so motivated. But not in my case.

Most think embryonic stem cell science is great because embryonic stem cells are so "pluripotent." People get very impressed with that medical nonsense, like being impressed with fractal mathematics for the evaluation of sand grains to find a pearl on the beach, and they swallowed it hook, line and sinker.

We Americans cannot afford the irony of our political left being unconsciously de facto anti-science and de facto anti-intellectual on the matter of stem cells.

So, absent religion, here is the science of embryonic stem cells stated as a doctor and not as a priest.

A primer on stem cell biology
The human embryo starts off as a single cell, called a zygote, which reproduces rapidly, producing a ball of cells (blastocyst).

The inside of the ball of cells (inner cell mass) contains multiple identical cells called embryonic stem cells, each of which can potentially build an entire baby with all its 220 (adult) post-birth cell types found in the human body from birth to death.

Therefore, natural embryonic stem cells are totally pluripotent (totipotent) because they can produce all 220 cell types. Embryonic stem cells are natural building stem cells, for the simple reason that they build an entire seven pound baby from a few identical natural building embryonic stem cells within nine months of pregnancy—an astronomical biological feat which modern science does not understand well.

Cancer
We all know how fast cancer grows.

Cancer can be defined as the overly rapid and uncontrolled multiplication of cells.

Importantly, no cancer known to modern medicine can grow so rapidly that it can produce a seven pound tumor from a single cell within nine months the way embryonic building stem cells can.

Natural building embryonic stem cells by virtue of their unique genetic activation are profoundly driven to build, build at a more frantic pace than any other cell type known to mankind.

Within the normal, natural surroundings within an intact embryo (its natural epigenetic milieu) this building cellular reproductive ferocity builds a human baby (embryogenesis, feto-genesis and fetal development), a complex biological process which employs very poorly understood DNA-related Herculean forces of nature which develop the human form (morphology).

The developmental forces of building an entire human baby from embryonic building stem cells is a highly mysterious process and modern medical science knows virtually nothing about how it works, except for elaborate growth stages (embryo and fetal microscopic descriptions) of what happens in this mysterious biologically powerful nine months of development (gestation).

What we don't know about embryo and fetal development is far greater than what we do know. Please recall with me what Albert Einstein said about our knowledge of all such matters: "We only know one thousandth of one percent of what nature has to teach us."

There is so much more to learn as there remain questions entirely unanswered in our primitive science of how DNA directs this well-orchestrated series of very rapid events of embryonic building stem cells during the nine months of pregnancy.

Yet, one thing we do know is that the cell multiplication rate of embryonic building stem cells is so fast that only the fastest growing cancer is comparable in cell multiplication speed.

When I was in medical school more than 30 years ago I learned about embryonic stem cells and adult stem cells. Therefore, stem cells are certainly not new. Soon thereafter a debate started to heat up about embryonic stem cells, which has since been heavily synthesized and readapted over the years with advanced biotechnology due to embryonic stem cells' lack of suitability to heal.

Embryonic stem cells are in fact … Cells-That-Do-Not-Heal.

Beside the fact that the science was faulty, the experimentation was objectionable to many because these scientifically ill-suited stem cells were being harvested from human embryos. Opponents of abortion were outraged, great pressure was brought to bear and the U.S. Food and Drug Administration issued its hysterical and ill-fated moratorium on all doctors from using treatments using any type of stem cells, including both adult stem cells (Healing Cells) as well as the awful embryonic stem cells (cells-that-do-not heal).

This is the current status of stem cell science in America; all stem cell treatments of any kind are effectively banned by the FDA in the U.S. because a very broad brushstroke was used to paint over a narrow abuse of medical science with a religious fervor.

As it turns out, we now know embryonic stem cells were the worst possible medical choice of which type of stem cells to study or to contemplate using on human patients. The original scientific thinking, before the 2000-DOCS discovered Healing Cells, was that because the embryo is just developing, embryonic stem cells would be more suitable for adapting (cellular plasticity of totipotency, extreme pleuripotency), and therefore, for healing injured tissues. **Once the 2000-DOCS found real natural healing cells, this idea became immediately obsolete.**

In fact, embryonic stem cells cause cancerous tumors to form when used in that manner, as an understanding of their scientific "baby building nature" would easily lead an intellectually free medical scientist to know.

Embryonic stem cells are clearly "cells-that-don't-heal" and "cells-that-build-cancer" outside of the embryo.

Embryonic stem cells are nature's building cells so they build ferocious cancers whenever they are taken out of the strong biologically controlled environment of a growing embryo.

Embryonic stem cells are highly inappropriate medically and are always dangerous for human stem cell treatments.

"Doctore, primum non nocere" (Doctor, first do

no harm)

(Hippocrates)

Patents Pending

So why were scientists so interested in stem cells that need a great deal of research, experimentation, synthesizing, bio-engineering and processing to be rendered usable as healing cells after the 2000-DOCS's discovery of natural Healing Cells?

Because American medicine has evolved within the framework of **the U.S. patent system**, and those who invest in medical breakthroughs expect profits in return, and they cannot generate those profits unless and until they can patent protect the technology to monopolize it.

Healing Cells are naturally occurring, so they are what they are, and do what they do, without any assistance from human ingenuity or innovation. They are natural; therefore, they cannot be patent protected easily in the U.S.

Embryonic stem cells, however, are a cancerous poison to the human body whenever they are taken outside of the strictly bio-controlled environment of a normal growing embryo and cannot be utilized until completely transformed by patentable processes.

Although they are medically inappropriate for human stem cell treatments, ironically, it is that very inappropriateness that renders embryonic stem cells so insanely suitable for medical U.S. patent protection.

That is why they lied to you, my fellow pro-science liberal Democrats.

To help the uninitiated better understand how American medical stem cell research has been turned on its ear, let's look at an analogy.

Acquafil

Let's say that we have the task of supplying drinking water to the masses.

The most efficient and healthy method is to set up at a relatively unspoiled and easily accessible site of a natural water source, construct a device to pump the water to a filtering site, bottle it, then deliver it to retail outlets for distribution.

Let's guess that we can deliver natural water, slightly processed for safety reasons, for around ten cents a gallon. We can sell it for 50 cents per gallon and make a sizeable profit, while keeping the price relatively affordable to all consumers.

If we are going to approach this hypothetical water problem analogously to the way medical research and the FDA is approaching Healing Cells, we need to ensure that the process or end product is patentable, so that no one else can produce it and sell it after we spend exorbitantly to develop it.

Therefore, we must begin with a substance that is not quite really water, but that can be turned into a water-like substance through a patentable process. We must also pretend that everyone is unaware that water is available in natural springs and that no one is smart enough to construct a well with a pump.

Ironically, this irrationality is the most befitting part of the allegory because that is just what America is doing with regard to natural Healing Cells.

Therefore, we will drill for, let's say, crude oil and extract it and ship it to processing facilities, where it will be filtered, synthesized and processed by a method we have obtained the patent for, until it is eventually transformed into a substance that is somewhat like water. We will call our product Acquafil, because our marketing research shows that people responded favorably to this name by 20 percent over all other names tried in our test series.

Acquafil will be obtainable through a doctor's prescription. The cost of Acquafil will be 20,000 dollars per gallon—which the pharmaceutical company will tell us is justified because Acquafil actually costs them 10,000 dollars to manufacture and, after all, they are entitled to recoup their development costs and make a reasonable profit for their stockholders, right?

Meanwhile, we ignore natural springs and wells the same way we are ignoring natural Healing Cells.

Except now, some doctors have gone out of the country, overseas, to test an idea that natural springs and wells will work much better than oil transformed into Acquafil.

Those who have invested so heavily in the patent protection for Acquafil must hope that the FDA will ban the use of all natural well and spring water in the U.S.

Also, we must convince people how unreasonable, unsafe and illegitimate these overseas natural springs and wells are all in an effort to preserve our lucrative Acquafil market here at home. Their greatest fear will be that someone will drill a well here in America and their lucrative monopoly will come crashing down in ruins.

Of course in our example, Aquafil represents embryonic stem cells converted by patentable processes into synthetic healing cells and natural springs and wells represent natural Healing Cells that can be easily, safely and inexpensively harvested and applied.

Indeed, this is the state of medical stem cell research in the U.S. now playing out in the medical research arena.

The former focus on embryonic stem cells

Embryonic totipotent building stem cells are never normally found in the human body after birth, because they are biologically too dangerous to reside there. These cells are entirely novel inside our bodies unrestrained by the powerful restrictions on their biological behavior that they would have inside a microscopic early embryo where they are normally found. Outside the surroundings (epigenetic milieu) of an intact embryo natural building embryonic stem cells demonstrate the exact biological activity that we identify in powerfully malignant cancer cells.

When taken out of their natural epigenetic surroundings totipotent embryonic building stem cells are ferociously growing malignant cancer cells.[37, 38, 39, 40]

So why are our country's scientists using up the puny amount of American research funding available in a medically unsound process of attempting to transform malignant cancer-forming building embryonic stem cells into healing cells when we have discovered the real deal, normal natural Healing Cells? And why are our taxes being spent by the NIH on embryonic stem cell research?

This hollow medical idea, an empty-suit idea, is reminiscent of trying to find a pearl in the sand, not by a simple, practical, rational, pro-science and pro-intellectual methodology of using a screen with holes smaller than the pearl, but a puffed up, hyped-up, impractical, highly technical notion of performing some masturbatory science of advanced mathematical calculus of fractal geometry on each grain of sand to turn these cells from building cells (their nature) to healing cells (not their nature), while ignoring cells that naturally heal. Did intellectual liberals get bamboozled by advanced math? Did you forget that scientists can be vastly impractical, clinically naïve and pie-in-the-sky foolish? They are not medical doctors forced to deal with medical reality daily with sick patients. They are people in labs with rats and test tubes who are impractically driving the future of American medicine without the help of real medical doctors who are not paying any attention to them because they are too busy saving lives with old, soon to be obsolete high-technology medical practices.

When our country's scholars are intellectually and economically enslaved by a patent scheme that is solely profit motivated, they end up working on wrong-minded projects using the wrong scientific focus and we end up with a problem that is life threatening, the current reality of embryonic scientists' direct-kills medical malpractice.

To take a cell type which has all the distinct characteristics of cancer when it is outside the embryo and attempt to use our infantile and crude knowledge of gene (DNA) activation and gene (DNA) functional mechanics to make healing cells from them is unworthy of a first year medical student's expected level of medical thought and skill.

Natural building embryonic stem cells and any type of synthetic, man-made healing cells derived from them or worse, derived from any unnatural synthetic embryonic building stem cells, are all unacceptably dangerous, and focusing on and researching their clinical use as healing cells **has and will continue to drastically delay** the development of the next great therapeutic paradigm in human medical history; Healing Cells.

The bitter truth is that embryonic stem cells are clearly by their nature cells-that-build-cancer and not Healing Cells in

any respect. That is profound medical truth that will pass the test of time, unlike the stem cell research goals of medically naïve and dangerous embryonic stem cell scientists who have Ph.D.s instead of M.D.s. How did our system allow for Ph.D.s to direct-kill any of us? They are lab scientists and clearly not medical doctors. They have never gotten out of bed at three in the morning to save a life. How did these non-medical people get the power to direct-kill us and our families? The medical system is very broken, just like our banks, and for many of the same reasons!

Our generation may never receive the great benefits available from the correct focus of research on the healing discovery of Healing Cells. Our country's scholars, medical scientists and physicians have lost their intellectual freedom, whether they realize it or not. But regaining and then retaining their intellectual freedom serves our country's best interests because collectively, our country's scholars and doctors represent a precious and valuable American resource, a great American national treasure, currently wrongly used.

This grand, national error will cost millions of lives and delay solving America's healthcare cost crisis to the tune of trillions of dollars every year until the error is reversed. The FDA and embryonic stem cell researchers are inadvertently causing vast "direct kills."

And like many direct-kills, the perpetrators are unaware of the effects of their actions until it is too late, like the ivory tower experts' faulty scientific evaluation of Dr. Jenner's cowpox vaccine, actions which likewise direct-killed many of their trusting contemporaries (including their own children) with smallpox?

Jenner's vaccine is a cautionary tale for today's ivory tower embryonic stem cell scientists and their financial and political backers who have already delayed Healing Cells science, and have in my professional opinion direct-killed many would-be successful patients already. In this book I formally charge them in the public square for their vast medical incompetence and medical malpractice.

The public has been calling for doctors to police themselves. I'm doing that now. It is malpractice; many have been hurt already by many medical professionals who continue to support this ridiculous wrong-minded medical science of embryonic stem cells, which are nothing but hurtful cancer cells whenever they are outside of the control of a normal embryo. Our current FDA supported ubiquitous scientific infatuation and hyper-focus with these cells in lieu of the more medically powerful natural Healing Cells is massive *de facto* malpractice.

Stem Cells

There is a group of cells within the 220 adult cells found in newborns that retain some ability to change into different cell types (pleuripotency); these are the post-birth stem cells (adult stem cells) found within bone marrow, some of which make up the Healing Cells organ system that functions naturally to heal the body from cradle to grave.

These Healing Cells are all adult stem cells because by definition they are post-birth cells (adult) and they can "stem" into other types of cells (pluripotent) to replace dying cells of our sick bodies. This has been happening since before we stood up on our hind legs.

These are the cells that make up the Healing Cells organ system within human bone marrow.

To be called Healing Cells, cells must **heal** naturally within their proper, natural, biological surroundings (normal epigenetic niche).

Only Healing Cells pass this critical test supporting their candidacy to be the appropriate focus of current stem cell medical research.

The actual cells that do the healing are not new to us, rather it is the healing process of these cells that is new; therefore, the healing process is what needs research. What needs to be explored is the healing process of Healing Cells, since it is the healing process that we did not know about before the work of the 2000-DOCS.

Embryonic building stem cells need to make other cell types (pluripotency) in order to build a baby, while Healing Cells make cells unlike themselves (pluripotency) in order to heal the body. Specifically, Healing Cells make cells unlike themselves at the point when they have reached the injured tissues, under the influence of cytokine attraction (chemo-attraction), at which time they transform (trans-differentiate) from Healing Cells into whatever cell types are needed to replace the dead and injured cells at the site of cellular injury from disease (see Addendum for details on these fascinating processes).

Embryonic building stem cells, on the other hand, are guided to transform into each of the 220 different post-birth cell types (adult) in a complex process of frantic cell reproduction (embryogenesis, fetogenesis and development), which takes nine months in humans (gestation).

Cell biologists have learned that the cell transformations (cellular trans-differentiations) of embryonic building stem cells are controlled largely by special hormone-like substances (cytokines).

Both natural and synthetic (bioengineered) embryonic building stem cells can be transformed by scientists into many different cell types by soaking them in certain cytokine soup recipes for cell growth cultures in predetermined sequences. There are already many earned intellectual properties and patents relating to the types and sequences of cytokine cell-culture recipes and procedures involved in these natural and unnatural categories of embryonic building stem cell transformations.

There will be many more.

Healing Cells are used in our overseas clinics essentially as they are found within nature. They are difficult to patent protect because they are natural and largely unchanged from their natural state when used clinically.

However, embryonic building stem cells when removed from an embryo cause deadly cancerous tumors if transplanted into a patient.

In fact, the scientific test used to determine the presence of embryonic building stem cells within a mouse belly cell culture is tumor formation (murine peritoneal living cell culture). **Therefore, everyone knows that embryonic building stem cells cannot be given to patients as they are found in nature because they will cause tumors.**

Embryonic building cancerous stem cells are perfectly **patentable** within our medical system because much patentable biotechnology is required in order to transform them from building cells, which invariably cause tumors, into cells that will heal, which are patentable but are synthetic, unnatural "healing" stem cells derived from embryonic building stem cells.

Researchers are going in reverse

It is my diagnosis that embryonic building stem cell investors are purposely ignoring the 2000-DOCS' discovery of the Healing Cells organ system merely because using this discovery would be very difficult to patent protect.

Furthermore, I believe that the embryonic building stem cell research industry is attempting to produce unnatural novel healing cells from dangerous embryonic building stem cells so they can have patentable healing cells with which to monopolize the coming stem cell therapeutic market. They are monetizing stem cell science in a harmful way while consciously ignoring a new discovery that is inexpensive, safer and far more likely to succeed.

The direct-kills in this terrible situation are all the patients who could be saved or relieved of grave suffering if it were not for the greedy embryonic stem cell scientists and their backers who are trying to hold up progress on natural healing cells until they can overcome the inborn cancer problem of embryonic stem cells, which they are far from accomplishing.

If this continues the American people will not see the cost of healthcare diminish, as it would through the development of treatments with natural Healing Cells.

Embryonic building stem cells make all the Healing Cells as well as the other post-birth (adult) cells. This is very important, so I'll reiterate:

Embryonic building stem cells make all cells including Healing Cells during normal embryologic development.

The shameful irony is that the American people are going to pay for intellectual property and patent fees to provide them with something we already have, namely, Healing Cells, ex-

cept these embryonic building stem cell-derived synthetic Healing Stem Cells will cost a fortune and allow the patent holders, the embryonic building stem cell investors, to use our well intentioned patent laws to control and continue to monopolize medical care in our country, which will perpetuate America's healthcare cost crisis. It's a Water vs. Aquafil contest in the making.

Induced pluripotent stem cell (iPSCs)

Another scheme of the embryonic building stem cell investors used to fool liberal intellectuals is to transform normal human body cells (somatic cells) into patentable manmade embryonic building stem cells by using a vector (often viruses or bacteria cell parts) to inject genetic material into them, converting them into a type of synthetic, manmade embryonic building stem cell called an induced pluripotent stem cell (iPSCs[41, 42, 43]).

This process seeks to avoid objections to embryonic building stem cell research based on abortion issues.

There will be huge patent costs needed to make these synthetic embryonic building stem cells safe for injection because these iPSCs also cause ferocious cancer just as do natural embryonic building stem cells when they are outside the protective environment of a growing embryo.

Then there will be the cost of research needed to transform these patented bio-engendered, embryonic building stem cells (iPCs) into synthetic unnatural healing stem cells, which will likewise be patented.

Then after all this cost we will be exactly where we are now, needing to do the research on the healing process protocols.

Roger M. Nocera, M.D.

Somatic cell nuclear transfer (SCNT)[44]

Yet another scheme attempts to create manmade embryonic building stem cells from normal skin cells instead of an embryo using technology called somatic cell nuclear transfer (SCNT), also known as therapeutic cloning. Before my fellow liberal Democrats get too impressed, please note that this manmade unnatural embryonic building stem cell from SCNT will never be a viable treatment option for the public because this technology suffers from prohibitively high costs of production plus all the cancer issues as well.

In order to make these synthetic embryonic building stem cells, which still have all the tumor and fierce malignancy biological behavior as natural embryonic building stem cells, a highly trained and skilled cell biologist (Ph.D. level) must meticulously take the nucleus out of a skin cell and place it into a donated human egg cell, by hand, under extreme microscopic conditions for each and every patient to be treated.

Since this is such a highly skilled, labor-intensive process, the costs of production will never decrease to an affordable level.

Moreover, this scheme will require a constant supply of healthy human egg cells which are obtained from women's ovaries in an expensive procedure that is invasive, risky and painful . . . and limited in availability.

After all these expenses of production there are still the costs to be paid for the patented processes needed to convert these synthetic tumor forming malignant embryonic building stem cells into healing cells that hopefully won't cause cancer.

As you can see, the embryonic building stem cell investors are not really against healing cell technology as long as it passes through their heavily patented embryonic building stem cell technology first, so that they can monopolize it through the patent system.

Embryonic building stem cells are totipotent by definition, which means that to be called an embryonic building stem cell, a stem cell must be potentially capable of creating an entire embryo, complete, from one cell.

Any totipotent cell will always cause cancers if ever it is taken out of the natural surroundings (epigenetic) of a growing embryo and injected into the natural surroundings within a patient.

Yes, scientists can create stem cell types from transforming embryonic building stem cells in the laboratory (cellular trans-differentiating), but these embryonic building stem cells transformations create "synthetic healing stem cells" that are either manufactured unnatural stem cell copies of what we already have and throw away, namely natural Healing Cells, or they are an unknown manmade patentable stem cell type. Embryonic building stem cells that are bio-engendered and transformed into patentable synthetic healing stem cells are no longer true natural and predictable cells. They are something else that have an infinite realm of variability and possible biological behaviors, which only years and years of exorbitantly expensive research could possibly uncover; a process, which is so expensive and time consuming as to be well beyond the life expectancy of the current generation, especially the baby-boomers.

This is just what the old paradigm investors want, since they are doing just fine selling synthetic drugs within the old therapeutic synthetic drug paradigm.

The largest, most profitable medical market for the foreseeable future within the U.S. is the baby boom generation, aging and already taking many expensive, patented, synthetic pharmaceuticals which are produced by those who profit in the current therapeutic paradigm, such as it is.

I'm Afraid It Just Isn't Totipotent Enough . . .

The built-in cellular healing organ system which repairs our bodies from cradle to grave uses Healing Cells which can transform into the different body cells that get injured and killed by disease.

Healing Cells, of course are not required to transform into every cell type the way embryonic building stem cells must do to build a whole baby, a fact which embryonic building stem cell researchers and investors hurl as an insult to the healing capacity of Healing Cells! And my lemming-like fellow liberal intellectuals swallow this medical science nonsense hook, line and sinker like this was an idea issued by the Pope!

It's like dismissing treatment with penicillin out of hand because it doesn't prevent pregnancy! The argument makes no sense, but when flung out within earshot of a lay audience it sounds authoritative and very scientific.

Observational science has taught us that cells that can make all 220 cell types, (totipotent stem cells) are always malignant outside the growing embryo's environment (epigenetic).

I know of no exceptions.

The natural cellular force of totipotency is biologically safe if and only if these cells are within a growing embryo's unique environment. Yet, the embryonic building stem cell advocates criticize the validity of Healing Cells healing potential because they claim that Healing Cells are not totipotent!

This is intellectual dishonesty to the point of lunacy.

It is entirely unnecessary for a healing stem cell to become a complete human—it need only become the type of cell it is sent to replace—heart tissue, intestinal tissue, brain tissue, muscle tissue, nerve tissue, vascular tissue, etc., which it obviously does quite well naturally.

That is the way our bodies have been healing and regenerating themselves since the first human, and for a researcher to pretend otherwise merely belies his true interests in the outcome—natural, easily obtainable Healing Cells vs. the insanity of unnatural, bio-engineered, patented and unsafe stem cells (50 cents/gal vs. $20,000/gal).

The FDA forbids doctors to begin the safest, quickest, least expensive pathway to develop Healing Cells therapeutics…that is our national problem.

Why then should we American citizens think for one minute that the FDA is functioning any more competently on this issue than the **Minerals Management Agency** was in regulating proper oil drilling safety in the Gulf of Mexico? Why would we think that? Because the FDA bureaucracy is so smart?

Apropos to this moment I would like to define the term "groupthink."

Groupthink is a type of thought exhibited by members of a group who try to minimize conflict and reach consensus without critically testing, analyzing and evaluating ideas. In groupthink, members of the group avoid promoting viewpoints outside the comfort zone of consensus thinking.

Groupthink helps medical scientists and FDA agents keep jobs that require groupthink philosophies by their employers. Groupthink is the mechanism that suppresses free thinking (innovation) in science in the manner referred to by President Eisenhower's words, ". . . the free university, historically the fountainhead of free ideas and scientific discovery has experienced a revolution in the conduct of research. Partly because of the huge costs involved, a contract becomes virtually a substitute for intellectual curiosity."

The world disposes of its afterbirth rich with Healing Cells as bio-waste and the FDA forbids the widespread use of the patient's own autologous Healing Cells, all the while the embryonic building stem cell scientists are trapped within a system which is forcing them to make patentable synthetic healing stem cells from natural and unnatural embryonic building stem cells. So, we trash the solution to our healthcare cost crisis and our country's scientists toil under the control of big money, groupthinking all the way, to invent artificially produced patentable embryonic building stem cells so that they can turn them into patentable synthetic healing stem cells so they can keep medicine expensive, patentable and profitable. Again, we are throwing out the natural, healthy, inexpensive spring water and investing heavily in the distant future of Aquafil. It is insanity.

Those who think they understand the medicine of stem cell science also wrongly think that President Bush's original ban on federally funded embryonic building stem cell research held up science; it did not.

The malignancy of totipotency of all types of embryonic building stem cells, a problem yet to be solved, created the holdup, a problem which still exists today. I cannot believe I am defending President Bush, with whom I agree on virtually nothing, because of his distinctly non-intellectual approach!

But let's face it, being an intellectual helps not if your facts are wrong!

Only groupthink spawned by self-interest can explain this behavior in scientists who must read the same valid research reports about the discoveries concerning Healing Cells that I have been presenting in this book. Moreover, this is their specialty, so not knowing or admitting the significance of these discoveries is not a viable explanation for their professional behavior. Yet keeping their jobs at the expense of their intellectual curiosity (and integrity) explains these medically illogical behaviors quite well.

Nature's healing cells, Healing Cells, are being largely ignored by the scientific and medical communities because they are all supported by big medical businesses, which would much rather continue inventing and selling synthetic drugs which are clearly very profitable than risk losing their gargantuan profits by investing in less expensive and more effective medical treatments that are unpatentable.

As indirectly warned against by President Eisenhower there are virtually no doctors or scientists in a position to decide which new medical therapies should be developed by research, unencumbered by the impact of patent-law economics and their investor-employers' profit goals. Our doctors are not deciding what therapies we will research; rather, non-doctor business people are deciding the focus of research and which therapies we will develop because they have all the embryonic stem cell scientists in their pockets.

This unfortunate arrangement has been the modus operandi of the American healthcare industry for at least the last five decades since Eisenhower issued his cautionary final speech as our President. This is the one and only reason for our dismal showing in the World Health Organization's 2000 report and the chief cause of our American healthcare cost crisis.

We have an industry run entirely by non-medical persons who are tied to big money investors who are completely captive by patent law, which powerfully favors unnatural therapies which do not work very well, exactly and precisely because they are so unnatural.

> "The prospect of domination of the nation's scholars
>
> by project allocations, and the power of money is ev-
>
> er present–and is gravely to be regarded . . ."
>
> (President Eisenhower)

The truth is that there is only one category of cell type, Healing Cells, that is worthy of the ponderously important medical research in this field now, at a time when funding is so scarce because of our nation's economy. Healing Cells, as the name purposely implies, are the only cells that exhibit the natural, intrinsic, human cellular healing process, a natural healing process only just discovered a few years ago, which will not be completely understood by medical scientists for decades to come.

Yet a complete understanding of the exact bio-mechanisms of these natural Healing Cells is not a prerequisite for their judicious therapeutic clinical use now in America, as we and others have been doing in overseas clinics for years.

Because Healing Cells are perfectly harmless, innocuous and totally benign, there need be no restrictions placed on our doctors' freedom to practice their profession by using these cells if that is the best medical course of action determined by the good judgment of highly trained physicians, as opposed to being restricted by the FDA to ignore the safety and promise of these treatments because of the government's uneducated, uninformed and special interest influenced edicts.

Our nation's doctors could provide to us the initial therapeutic benefits, which are harmlessly available within our own (autologous) Healing Cells now, today, at a much lower cost than currently available treatments were it not for the FDA legal restrictions placed upon our American physicians' freedom to prescribe them.

This makes no practical sense since it is a fact that a patient's own Healing Cells (autologous cells) have an undeniably favorable safety profile.

We have weakened our American culture by failing to honor the intellectual freedom of those who have dedicated their lives to the discovery of scientific medical truth . . . our nation's medical scholars, our physicians, who collectively represent a vitally important but finite American resource, which will be much needed if we are to solve the challenges of 21st Century life.

The government could initiate this paradigm shift for mankind by simply getting the FDA to declare autologous Healing Cells legal for doctors to prescribe; the rest would happen automatically.

Doctors would then be free to add these harmless cells into their treatment regimens.

A central database could be inexpensively set up to coordinate the results from doctors all over the country who would be treating patients with their own Healing Cells.

New Healing Cells protocols would soon emerge without the prohibitive expense of traditional formal research and exorbitant patent defense costs, which no one will pay for because these cells are so natural as to be difficult if not impossible to patent-defend in our legal system.

We need to study Healing Cells now before any foolish and dangerous attempts are made to re-engineer nature before we know how it works, which is the current plan of the embryonic building stem cell patent holders, the biggest players in the entire stem cell space.

The sitting President and Congress could create a Healing Cells "Manhattan Project" to produce natural and unpatentable Healing Cells protocols for legal treatments before the investors can produce patentable unnatural ones from embryonic building stem cells, which will delay our needed medical paradigm shift while keeping our healthcare costs in the stratosphere.

Doing nothing will give the embryonic building stem cell investors time to evolve their patent-heavy embryonic building stem cell transformation trick to manufacture bastardized, patentable synthetic unnatural and maybe "healing" cells that hopefully will not retain any of the cancerous totipotency within the transformation cultures, an accomplishment very far from achievable, which is why after all the American hype about the power of stem cells we have no treatments available with the wrong-minded embryonic stem cell focus scientific approach (fractal geometry of sand grains).

Advocating embryonic stem cell research over Healing Cells research is simply an unnecessary, abhorrent, financial play on the American people, a play which parallels the hedge fund derivative mortgage security banking scandal the world just experienced from similar self-serving, shallow-minded profiteering.

I have sent copies of this book to the President, Vice President, and members of the U.S. Congress in both the Senate and the House of Representatives.

I have sent copies to many other public figures as well, in the hope of getting this critical and timely message out to those who are empowered and charged by their constituents to facilitate the development of the most crucial medical discovery in human history once it is presented to them.

I am asking everyone who reads Cells That Heal to write a letter to the President and their government congressional representatives, urging them to read the copies they were sent and to immediately and positively act upon this important information.

To our detriment, our country's physicians have been kept in the dark about this new medical scientific discovery; therefore, after reading this book it would be helpful if you could give your copy to your personal physician and urge him or her to read it.

Proceeds from sales of this book will
be donated to a charitable foundation
which I have created called FACTs,
The Foundation for the Advancement
of Cells-that-heal Therapeutics.

We have inherited one of the most profoundly transformative moments in human medical history. A paradigm shift in human therapeutics is at hand, which our actions could trigger and assist. Whatever our national problems, be they domestic or foreign, the outcomes are bound to be better for us if Americans become healthier, especially if we can accomplish that great task while simultaneously spending a fraction of our current exorbitant and soon to become prohibitive national healthcare expense.

"The medical industry is like a large
tree with many branches. What most
people have lost sight of is that the
trunk of the tree upon which all the
branches depend is scientific medical
research."

If you have questions about this book and Healing Cells or our foundation FACTs

please visit our website at http://www.CellsThatHeal.com

ADDENDUM

HOW HEALING CELLS WORK

"The art of medicine consists in amusing the patient while nature cures the disease."

(Voltaire)

Cells

One of my professors in graduate physiology once told our class to think of human cells as miniature human beings. This turned out to be very insightful—a medical information pearl. It is a scientifically accurate and most helpful way to think about cells because both individual human beings and individual human cells share many of the same traits:

- both are dynamic, active and living; alive

- both eat food and make usable energy with it;

- both produce and eliminate waste;

- both breath oxygen and make carbon dioxide;

- both reproduce;

- both have parents, siblings and offspring;

- both have parts that are devoted to specialized functions;

- both contain our total identical DNA genetic codes which guide these innate activities in ways we know little about;

- both have a kind of intelligence;

- both are either male or female;

- both are interdependent with their fellows;

- both differentiate into specialized individuals capable of specialized performance that helps its neighbor's survival and wellbeing.

- both get sick;

- both heal;

- both are born;

- both die; and

- we have vital measurements to test the level of health of both.

Also, in a manner that we do not completely understand, we know that humans, as all living creatures, are quite simply a reflection of our cells; we mirror them and they mirror us. In some way or another, we are our cells. But most importantly, we are as healthy, no more or less, than the collective health of our body's cells, the smallest fundamental units of our living being. No medical doctor would argue with that.

Well established medical biology

Before discussing the momentous discovery of Healing Cells in greater depth, which is relatively new science not yet well disseminated even to most doctors, let's first review some well-established conventional medical science of human cell function so that you may draw a realistic scientific comparison between the two.

This introduction will help you understand the newer science of Healing Cells, which is so intricate and brilliantly elegant that it might seem somewhat mystical, or even miraculous at first. I assure you, these are real, natural processes which have been in place for millions of years and meticulously observed and documented by hard science for many decades. As you will see, many key aspects contributing to the healing functions of Healing Cells have already been well established in biology and medical science as fact, long ago.

Routine appendicitis

Here's an example of how some cells work —these facts have been well known for decades.

If you go to the hospital with appendicitis, one of your doctor's concerns will be that you may have developed a bag of infectious pus (an abscess) in your abdomen.

If you do develop one of these nasty bags of germs and it bursts open into the lining of your abdominal organs (peritoneum), infection from the germs could spread very fast throughout your whole abdominal cavity (bacterial peritonitis) and from there they can easily spread into the blood in vast numbers (overwhelming septicemia), which can readily kill you by causing your blood pressure to drop too low to support your body's vital functions (sepsis induced third spacing of body fluids, systemic hypovolumemia, vascular hypotension, multi-organ hypoperfusion, generalized multi-organ ischemic pathophysiology, acute renal failure from systemic hypotension, acute tubular necrosis, multi-organ system failure and death by overwhelming septic shock).

This is why appendicitis, when it forms a pus germ bag (an abscess), which happens quite often, can be so potentially dangerous that doctors are and should be concerned about appendicitis whenever it occurs and react to it as a potentially rapidly progressive acute disease requiring relatively emergent surgery to remove the pus-producing problem ("never let the sun set on an abscess").

Pus formation in appendicitis, which we will walk through now, illustrates a complex and well understood natural cell process of enormous medical scientific importance in the Healing Cell discovery.

The cause of appendicitis (etiologic pathophysiology)
There is a little worm-shaped, tube-like pouch called the appendix, which extends from the end part of the large bowel (the cecum).

The first thing that happens to trigger the condition called appendicitis (pathogenesis) is that the appendix's worm-like pouch gets clogged up by something passing by in the solid waste material of the bowel (mechanical appendiceal obstruction by fecal debris).

The clog, like all clogs in any biological-tube anatomical structure, backs things up and creates a lot of back-pressure within the tube-like pouch. That harsh backpressure really messes everything up where the appendix cells live (disrupts vital local tissue homeostasis). This backpressure itself directly causes damage to the cells of the appendix. It's like hitting and smashing them over the head; and among many other problems, it causes a breakdown of the natural barriers normally preventing the infection of the deep appendix cell neighborhood from incursion and attack by nearby large bowel (symbiotic fecal E. coli and others).

When the cells of the appendix suffer enough damage from back pressure and infection they start dying in droves. When appendix cells die, as when all cells die suddenly, they break apart (perturbation of cell membrane integrity, disruption of the cell's sodium-potassium pump, lost osmotic regulation, etc.) and spill all their insides, all their appendix cell-guts, all their vital cell contents into the surrounding neighborhood of fellow appendix cells (appendix organ tissues), analogous to soldiers spilling their blood when they get hit and killed on a battlefield.

More and more appendix cells die from the backpressures of the clogged pouch, and they suffer from these disturbing effects upon their previously happy appendix cell neighborhood (appendix tissues), which is now being further ruined by an invasion of large bowel germs (fecal E. coli and others). All this destruction causes more and more appendix cells to likewise die and break open, spilling out more appendix cell guts onto the worsening cell battlefield. Cell death starts to spread like an epidemic throughout the appendix cell neighborhood where the appendix cells were happily living before the pouch got clogged up.

Now things begin to happen that are triggered one after the other, with one event leading to the next, in a biological chain reaction of normal physiologic events that produce the bag of germs and dead soldier appendix cells (a cascade of natural biochemical reactions triggered in sequence from endocrine and paracrine local and distant physiologic and pathophysiologic events leading to pus formation).

Natural human drugs (cytokines)

Among the contents spilling out of the broken appendix cells are very active chemical substances called cytokines (si-tuh-kīns), which are very special because they cause things to happen (hormonal triggers) not only at the site of the injured appendix cells' neighborhood (cytokine induced local tissue hormonal paracrine effects) but also cause important things to happen far away from the injury, elsewhere in the body (cytokine induced distant tissue hormonally triggered physiologic events).

As more appendix cells die these active chemical substances (cytokines) begin to accumulate and become highly concentrated in and around the appendix cells' neighborhood.

These active chemical substance concentrations (local tissue cytokine levels) rise ever higher from more and more cell death-induced cell guts spillage until the local appendix cell neighborhood gets so filled up with dying appendix cell guts (cytokines) that these chemicals spill over from the appendix cell neighborhood into the blood, which is circulating nearby, increasing their concentration within the blood, a measurable event (measurable specific cytokine blood levels).

The active chemical substances (Granulocyte Stimulating Factor cytokines), which are now increasing within the blood, act as a chemical signal that travels through the blood circulation throughout the body, reaching the bone marrow where they (hormonally) signal stimulation of certain bone marrow tissue cells (granulocytic cell line of hematopoietic adult stem cells) to produce and release into the blood vast numbers of specialized cells called white blood cells (neutrophils).

As this process continues over the next few hours to days, the white blood cell concentration in the blood will increase way above normal range. Your doctor will know this because she will order a test called a white blood cell count (a white count, neutrophil blood count). The white blood cell count will reveal these rapidly produced massive numbers of white blood cells pouring into the blood in ever increasing numbers from hormonally activated bone marrow.

The bone marrow is producing them and sending them into the blood as fast as it can under the influence and stimulation of rising appendix cell guts (cytokines like GCSF) also pouring into the blood from the poor appendix cells' deaths (an elevated white count with a left shift caused by rapidly elevated blood levels of granulocyte stimulating factor cytokine blood levels coming from dying appendix cells, which hormonally stimulate hematopoietic granulocyte precursor adult stem cells to produce neutrophils in bone marrow tissue).

The cell attraction trick (cytokine chemotaxis)

The second function of these active chemical substances (cytokines) spilling out from dying appendix cells is to attract (hormonally) the white blood cells (neutrophil granulocytes) as they pass by within the circulating blood, which causes them to be pulled toward the problem and accumulate inside the appendix cell neighborhood very rapidly (pulled in the direction of increasing cytokine concentration gradients).

This process is called "chemo-attraction" or "chemotaxis," which attracts white blood cells to cytokines as if by magic, but it's not; rather it's well understood, old, hard medical science.

This hormonal attraction (chemo-attraction or chemotaxis) of white blood cells to these accumulating active chemical substances is so powerful that a bag of white pus (an abscess) may begin to accumulate in and around the appendix cell neighborhood, becoming the size of a fist or largeru within a matter of a few days, composed largely of all those white blood cells and dead appendix cell soldiers.

That represents a lot of cells, many millions of cells, in fact.

These active chemical substances spilled from the dying appendix cells (inflammatory interleukin cytokines, tumor necrosis factor-alpha cytokine, GCSF, etc.) also open holes within the blood vessels (increased vascular permeability) so that the white blood cells can pass more easily from the blood compartment into the appendix cell neighborhood as they pass by within the blood in elevated concentrations.

White blood cells swallow up the germs
The vitally important function of this series of natural physiological events, without which we would die from trivial infections, is to generate a coordinated, rapid and overwhelming production and delivery of white blood cells that function to swallow up and kill the infecting bacteria (germicidal cellular phagocytosis) and remove the dead cells, in this case dead appendix cells.

This is what white blood cells do.

So the cell damage from a clogged up appendix triggers a series of events, controlled by active chemical substances (cytokines) spilling out of broken appendix cells, which automatically stimulate the production and release of white blood cells from bone marrow tissue (hematopoietic adult stem cells), which elevates the white blood cell count and also attracts them to the very site where they are needed to kill and swallow up the invading germs and to clean up debris from the dead, broken appendix tissue cells.

Released cytokines from injured appendix cells generate an efficient chemical signaling system, which uses the blood circulatory system as a delivery tool to the bone marrow to hormonally stimulate the production and release of millions of white blood cells into the blood circulation, which we can measure in our medical laboratories.

The blood now rich in white blood cells in turn delivers the white blood cell fighting army to exactly where it is needed at the site of infection. Then the chemo-attraction forces attract the white blood cell army to exactly the point of cell injury and bacteria wherever it might be within the body. [2, 3]

Fascinating, isn't it?

These are indisputable medical facts that medical scientists have been aware of for many decades. (Classic cytokine induced inflammatory cellular pathophysiology)

The Healing Cells organ system
What follows is one of those monumental, hundred-year discoveries of nature which change humanity forever.

When there is damage of any kind in the body for whatever reason, cells get injured and die. That is what diseases and injuries do.

Just as in the case of appendicitis, when cells die they break open and spill their contents including their special chemical substances (cytokines) into the surrounding cell neighborhood where they were living before they got hurt (native organ tissues).

As these active chemical substances (cytokines) accumulate in their tissue neighborhood they spill over into the blood, just as they did in appendicitis. The increase of released cytokines from injured cells can be measured in the medical laboratory (specific cytokine blood levels)

The elevated blood levels of these active chemical substances (injured cell released cytokines), are carried as hormonal messengers through the circulation to be delivered to all other parts of the body.

When the cytokines get to the bone marrow they hormonally trigger the bone marrow tissue to produce Healing Cells from specialized cells in the bone marrow (adult stem cell precursors to various cell lineages leading to specific Healing Cells phenotypes such as CD34 +, EPCs, mesenchymal) and release them into the blood in large numbers (many millions), whereby the Healing Cells blood count increases and can be scientifically measured exactly like an elevated white blood cell count in routine appendicitis. Next, just as in the case of white blood cells in pus formation, the Healing Cells are attracted to the injured tissue's high cytokine concentration by the process of chemo-attraction.[26, 27, 28, 29, 30, 31, 32, 33, 35]

Just as white blood cells are attracted into the sick appendix cell neighborhood when the appendix gets clogged up in appendicitis, the Healing Cells are sent out to help. Chemical substances (cell specific cytokines spilled by injured cells) also hormonally signal the local blood vessels to enlarge (vasodilatation) to bring more Healing Cells rich blood to the cell injury site. These chemical substances (cell specific cytokines) hormonally signal the development of holes in the local blood vessel walls (increased vascular permeability), which aid the Healing Cells in accessing the site of injury from the blood, where they begin to accumulate in vast numbers by the hormonal attraction forces of the cytokines (chemotaxis) exactly where they are needed precisely as white blood cells do in appendicitis. There is no new medical science here.

The new big thing

The Healing Cells are further influenced (hormonally) by the local cytokine substances at the site of cell injury to transform into the type of cells that are needed to rebuild and repair tissue damage by replacement of the cells in a process well known called cellular trans-differentiation—cells transforming into the different types of cells. If the cell damage happens to be located in the heart - a heart attack (ischemic myocardial infarction) - then the Healing Cells will transform into heart cells (cardiomyocytes) to replace the dead and dying heart cell units under the influence of dying heart cell cytokine substance release. Whereas, if the damage is within the brain (ischemic brain infarct), then the cytokines from the damaged brain cells will signal the Healing Cells to transform into brain cells (neurons) when they arrive on the cytokine rich scene of brain tissue damage, created by brain cell death and brain cell content spillage.

Whatever the tissue that is damaged from whatever injury or disease process that may have occurred anywhere in the body from whatever cause, the resultant cytokine substance spillage from broken, injured cells will signal the hormonal stimulation of just the right types and combination of the different Healing Cells to be produced and released into the blood circulation from the bone marrow.

The Healing Cells are then delivered via the blood to the injured cells' neighborhood (organ tissues) where they accumulate by the biochemical attraction they have for cytokines. All of the different types of tissues in the body have their own cellular identity, an identity which is reflected in the types of active chemical cytokine substances they release when injured and killed. Healing Cells are chemically triggered (hormonally) to transform into the appropriate cell type (cellular trans-differentiation) for cell unit replacement within the injured cell neighborhood (homing followed by cell trans-differentiation and engraftment).

This natural process is staggeringly beautiful and efficient.

An analogy
This process could be compared with a large collection of orchards, growing and thriving next to one another.

There would be apple trees, plum trees, pear trees, peach trees, cherry trees, etc.

Think of Healing Cells in this way—if some of the trees in one of the orchards were damaged, let's say in the peach orchard, the body would send out a plain wooden branch or stump (Healing Cells), and not until after it arrived among the peach trees would the pollen (specific cytokines) from the destroyed and remaining peach trees signal to the stump how it should rapidly develop and transform.

Having received the hormonal signature of the surrounding trees from their pollen, the stump would quickly transform into a peach tree, growing peach tree branches, blossoms and fruit.

Similar branches or stumps would arrive on the scene and transform, and before you knew it the peach tree orchard would be filled with trees and fruit, just as it was before the injury.

We now know that this magnificent process is how our bodies repair injuries caused by wounds or diseases.

Another big new thing, natural drugs-that-heal

When injury from disease of any kind hurts and kills cells, Healing Cells get produced and released into the blood, and "home" to the injured tissue. They transform themselves into the needed type of rebuilding cells (trans-differentiate[6]) to replace dead and injured cells. Then they also do something that is, like everything else in this new medical arena, profoundly amazing:

In response to cytokine stimulation Healing Cells release their own active natural therapeutic drugs (various active cytokines of their own). The cytokines of dead cells stimulate Healing Cells that arrive on the injury scene to become cytokine factories, pouring natural cytokine, powerfully biologically active natural drugs into our blood, measurably raising their blood levels. These cytokine natural substances are known to have healing effect, which scientists call "trophic effects." [7, 8] The cytokine released by Healing Cells favorably affect the surrounding cells, those that are damaged and even the undamaged tissue cells, locally and in other parts of the body, which greatly aid the body's healing process (trophic effects). The hormonal cytokine trophic effects cause healing in complex multi-factorial synergistic ways that medical scientists have only just begun to become conscious of and understand.

Roger M. Nocera, M.D.

This healing organ system is working every second of every day, from cradle to grave, keeping our bodies repaired by cell replacement and their own natural medicine cabinet composed of a series of natural therapeutic drugs.

ENDNOTES

1. Deb et al Circulation. 2003;107:1247.
2. Antibiot Chemother. 1974;19:409-20.
3. Immunology. 1969 Feb;16(2):231-9.
4. Orlic et al, Nature 2001 Apr 5; 410(6829) : 701-5.
5. Deb et al Circulation. 2003;107:1247.
6. J Cell Sci. 2002 Dec 1;115 (Pt23): 4617-28.
7. J of Cellular Biochem Vol 98 Issue 5 pages 1076-1084.
8. J. Clin. Invest. 114(6): 765-774 (2004).
9. Deb et al Circulation. 2003;107:1247.
10. Dunac et al, Neurol 2007 Mar, 254 (3) :327- 32.
11. Levesque et al, Handb Exp pharmacol. 2007; (180).
12. Grundmen et al Clin Ros Cardiolo 2007 Aug 13.
13. Ibid.
14. J Gerontol A Biol Sci Med Sci. 2006 Feb;61(2):190-5.
15. Hepatology Vol 36 Issue 5 Pages 1295-1297.
16. Mol Hum Reprod. 2003 Aug;9(8):497-502.
17. Hematol 2005, 33:165-172.
18. J Leukoc Biol 2004,75:314-323.
19. Blood 1997, 90:85-96.
20. Leukemia 1998, 12:728-734.
21. Blood 2004, 104:2010-2019.
22. Blood 2003, 101:168-172.
23. Stem Cells 2006.. Kern S, et al Comparative Analysis of Mesenchymal Stem Cells from Bone Marrow, Umbilical Cord Blood or Adipose Tissue.
24. Blood. 2003 Jul 15; 102(2):517-20.
25. Reprod Biomed Online 2008 Jun;16(6):898-905, Ichim et al.
26. Dev Dyn 2007 Dec;236(12):3321-31.
27. Circulation. 2003;107:461–8.
28. Cytotherapy. 2002;4:521–5.
29. Ann N Y Acad Sci. 2003;996:152–7.
30. Cell. 2003;114:763–76.
31. Exp Cell Res 2006, 312:2454-246.
32. J Exp Med 2004, 200:123-135.
33. Proc Natl Acad Sci U S A 2006, 103:7801-7806.
34. Cell Prolif 2005, 38:245-255.
35. Exp Cell Res 2004, 295:350-359.
36. Cell Prolif 2004,37:295-306.
37. Results Probl Cell Differ. 1980;11:265-74.
38. Nat Biotechnol 2000;18(4):399-404, 2000;18(5):559.
39. Science 1998;282(5391):1145-1147, 1998;282 (5395):1827.
40. J Cereb Blood Flow Metab 2003;23(7):780-785.
41. Nature. 2009 Jul 2;460(7251):49-52.
42. Curr Protoc Stem Cell Biol. 2009 Jun;Chapter 4:Unit 4A.2.

43. Biol. 2009 Jul;29(7):1100-3. Epub 2009 May 7.
44. Sheng Li Ke Xue jin Zhan 2009 Apr; 40(2) : 101-5.
45. Bone Marrow Transplant. 2009 Mar;43(5):417-22.
46. Cell Transplant. 2006;15(8-9):675-87.
47. Presse Med. 2005 Feb 26;34(4):311-8. Review. French.
48. Zhongguo Shi Yan Xue Ye Xue Za Zhi. 2005 Feb;13(1):30-4. Chinese.
49. Expert Opin Biol Ther. 2003 Apr;3(2):215-25. Review.
50. Exp Hematol. 2000 Jul;28(7):858-70.
51. Bone Marrow Transplant. 2000 Jun;25(11):1165-74.
52. Bone Marrow Transplant. 1999 Jun;23(11):1177-81.
53. Leuk Lymphoma. 1996 Oct;23(3-4):305-11.
54. Orlic et al, Nature 2001 Apr 5; 410(6829) : 701-5.
55. Deb et al Circulation. 2003;107:1247.
56. Bone Marrow Transplant. 2009 Mar;43(5):417-22.
57. Cell Transplant. 2006;15(8-9):675-87.
58. Presse Med. 2005 Feb 26;34(4):311-8. Review. French.
59. Zhongguo Shi Yan Xue Ye Xue Za Zhi. 2005 Feb;13(1):30-4. Chinese.
60. Expert Opin Biol Ther. 2003 Apr;3(2):215-25. Review.
61. Exp Hematol. 2000 Jul;28(7):858-70.
62. Bone Marrow Transplant. 2000 Jun;25(11):1165-74.
63. Bone Marrow Transplant. 1999 Jun;23(11):1177-81.
64. Leuk Lymphoma. 1996 Oct;23(3-4):305-11.
65. Semin Nucl Med. 2009 Jan;39(1):27-35. Review.
66. Semin Nucl Med. 2009 Jan;39(1):27-35. Review.
67. Schonberger S, Niehues T, Meisel R, Bernbeck B, Laws HJ, Kogler G.
68. Klin Padiatr 2004, 216:356-363.
69. Bone Marrow Transplant 2006, 38:421-426.
70. Eur J Haematol 2006, 77:46-50.
71. Bone Marrow Transplant 1998, 22 Suppl 1:S76-7.
72. Bone Marrow Transplant 2001, 27:693-701.
73. Hematology Am Hematol Educ Program. 2004:354-71 Stem Cell Transplants.
74. Lancet 1939, 2:1263.
75. Lancet 2003, 361:678-679.
76. J Am Coll Surg 2005, 200:557-563.
77. Clin Exp Obstet Gynecol 2006, 33:99-104.
78. Clin Exp Obstet Gynecol 2006, 33:39-43.
79. Clin Exp Obstet Gynecol 2006, 33:28-33.
80. Malar J 2006, 5:20.
81. Clin Exp Obstet Gynecol 2006, 33:117-121.
82. Eur J Gynaecol Oncol 2006, 27:286-290.
83. Biol Blood Marrow Transplant 2005, 11:149-160.
84. Klin Padiatr 2004, 216:356-363.
85. Bone Marrow Transplant 2006, 38:421-426.

86. Eur J Haematol 2006, 77:46-50.
87. Bone Marrow Transplant 1998, 22 Suppl 1:S76-7.
88. Bone Marrow Transplant 2001, 27:693-701.
89. Hematology Am Hematol Educ Program. 2004.354-71.
90. Journal of Translational Medicine 2007, 5:8
91. JAMA 2004; 292;75-80.
92. Blood 1996, 88:4390-4395.
93. Proc Natl Acad Sci U S A 1996, 93:705-708.
94. Lancet 2004, 364:179-182.
95. J Cell Sci 2005, 118:1559-1563.
96. Hepatology 2002, 36:1295-1297.
97. Lancet 2001, 358:2034-2038.
98. Jama 2004, 292:75-80.
99. Biotechniques 2003, 34:242-244.
100. Curr Opin Obstet Gynecol 2003, 15:195-199.
101. Biochem Biophys Res Commun 2004, 325:961-967.
102. Stem Cells 2005, 23:1443-1452.
103. J Clin Endocrinol Metab. 2005 Sep;90(9):5309-12.
104. Curr Opin Investig Drugs 2006, 7:473-481.
105. Stem Cells 2006, 24:1620-1626.
106. Cytotherapy 2005, 7:368-373.
107. Transfus Apher Sci 2004, 30:153-156.
108. Haematologica 2003, 88:958-960.
109. Lancet Vol 351, Issue 9113, 9 May 1998, Pages 1379-1387.
110. N Engl J Med. 1993 Jan 28;328(4):221-7.
111. JAMA. 1991 Dec 18;266(23):3289-94.
112. CMAJ. 2002 Apr 30;166(9):1169-79 Barnett HJ, et al,
113. Neurology 2005;65;794-801.
114. Stroke Cerebrovasc Dis. 2009 Jul-Aug;18(4):277-80.
115. Circulation. 1995 May 1;91(9):2325-34.
116. West J Med. 1982 April; 136(4): 295–308.
117. J Am Coll Cardiol, 1984; 3:114-128.
118. Circulation, Vol 82, 1629-1646.
119. N Engl J Med 1988 Aug 11 319 366-368.
120. Lancet. 1994 Aug 27;344(8922):563-70.
121. Deb et al Circulation. 2003;107:1247.
122. Dwight D. Eisenhower's Farwell Address to the Nation January 17, 1961.
123. Deb et al Circulation. 2003;107:1247.

Made in the USA
Charleston, SC
13 October 2011